Clinical Update on Adult and Pediatric Gastrointestinal Stromal Tumor

Guest Editors

JONATHAN C. TRENT, MD, PhD
SHREYASKUMAR R. PATEL, MD

HEMATOLOGY/ONCOLOGY CLINICS OF NORTH AMERICA

www.hemonc.theclinics.com

February 2009 • Volume 23 • Number 1

SAUNDERS an imprint of ELSEVIER, Inc.

W.B. SAUNDERS COMPANY
A Division of Elsevier Inc.

1600 John F. Kennedy Blvd. ● Suite 1800 ● Philadelphia, PA 19103-2899

http://www.theclinics.com

HEMATOLOGY/ONCOLOGY CLINICS OF NORTH AMERICA Volume 23, Number 1
February 2009 ISSN 0889-8588, ISBN 13: 978-1-4377-0486-0, ISBN 10: 1-4377-0486-7

Editor: Kerry Holland

Hematology/Oncology Clinics (ISSN 0889-8588) is published bimonthly by Elsevier Inc., 360 Park Avenue South, New York, NY 10010-1710. Months of issue are February, April, June, August, October, and December. Business and Editorial Offices: 1600 John F. Kennedy Blvd., Suite 1800, Philadelphia, PA 19103-2899. Customer Service Office: 11830 Westline Industrial Drive, St. Louis, MO 63146. Periodicals postage paid at New York, NY and additional mailing offices. Subscription prices are $283.00 per year (domestic individuals), $439.00 per year (domestic institutions), $141.00 per year (domestic students/residents), $321.00 per year (Canadian individuals), $537.00 per year (Canadian institutions) $382.00 per year (international individuals), $537.00 per year (international institutions), and $191.00 per year (international and Canadian students/residents). International air speed delivery is included in all *Clinics* subscription prices. All prices are subject to change without notice. **POSTMASTER:** Send address changes to *Hematology/Oncology Clinics of North America*, 11830 Westline Industrial Drive, St. Louis, MO 63146. Customer Service (orders, claims, online, change of address): Elsevier Periodicals Customer Service, 11830 Westline Industrial Drive, St. Louis, MO 63146. Tel: 1-800-654-2452 (U.S. and Canada). Fax: 314-523-5170. E-mail: journalscustomerservice-usa@elsevier.com (for print support); journalsonlinesupport-usa@elsevier.com (for online support).

Reprints. For copies of 100 or more, of articles in this publication, please contact the Commercial Reprints Department, Elsevier Inc., 360 Park Avenue South, New York, New York 10010-1710; Tel.: 212-633-3813, Fax: 212-462-1935, E-mail: reprints@elsevier.com.

Hematology/Oncology Clinics of North America is covered in *MEDLINE/PubMed (Index Medicus), EMBASE/ Excerpta Medica, and BIOSIS.*

Printed and bound by CPI Group (UK) Ltd, Croydon, CR0 4YY

Transferred to Digital Print 2011

Contributors

GUEST EDITORS

JONATHAN C. TRENT, MD, PhD
Assistant Professor, Department of Sarcoma Medical Oncology, The University of Texas
M.D. Anderson Cancer Center, Houston, Texas

SHREYASKUMAR R. PATEL, MD
Center Medical Director, Sarcoma Center; Professor, Department of Sarcoma Medical
Oncology, The University of Texas M.D. Anderson Cancer Center, Houston, Texas

AUTHORS

EDDIE K. ABDALLA, MD
Associate Professor, Department of Surgical Oncology, The University of Texas,
M.D. Anderson Cancer Center, Houston, Texas

RINKI AGARWAL, MBBS
Fellow, Department of Medicine, Clinical Genetics, Memorial Sloan-Kettering Cancer
Center, New York, New York

RONY AVRITSCHER, MD
Assistant Professor, Department of Diagnostic Radiology, The University of Texas
M.D. Anderson Cancer Center, Houston, Texas

PIYAPORN BOONSIRIKAMCHAI, MD
Postdoctoral Fellow, Department of Diagnostic Radiology, The University of Texas
M.D. Anderson Cancer Center, Houston, Texas

UMER I. CHAUDHRY, MD
Hepatobiliary Service, Memorial Sloan-Kettering Cancer Center, New York, New York

VISHNU CHINTALGATTU, PhD
Research Scientist, Department of Cardiology, The University of Texas M.D. Anderson
Cancer Center, Institute of Biosciences and Technology, Houston, Texas

HAESUN CHOI, MD
Professor, Department of Diagnostic Radiology, The University of Texas M.D. Anderson
Cancer Center, Houston, Texas

RONALD P. DeMATTEO, MD
Hepatobiliary Service, Memorial Sloan-Kettering Cancer Center, New York, New York

S. SERDAR DOGAN, MD
Section of Ophthalmology, Department of Head and Neck Surgery, The University
of Texas M.D. Anderson Cancer Center, Houston, Texas

BITA ESMAELI, MD
Associate Professor, Section of Ophthalmology, Department of Head and Neck Surgery, The University of Texas M.D. Anderson Cancer Center, Houston, Texas

SUZANNE GEORGE, MD
Instructor of Medicine, Harvard Medical School; Clinical Director, Center for Sarcoma and Bone Oncology, Dana-Farber Cancer Institute, Boston, Massachusetts

SANJAY GUPTA, MD
Associate Professor, Department of Diagnostic Radiology, The University of Texas M.D. Anderson Cancer Center, Houston, Texas

JASON L. HORNICK, MD, PhD
Department of Pathology, Brigham and Women's Hospital, Harvard Medical School, Boston, Massachusetts

KATHERINE A. JANEWAY, MD
Instructor of Pediatrics, Department of Pediatrics, Harvard Medical School; Attending Physician, Dana Farber Cancer Institute, Children's Hospital, Boston, Massachusetts

AARIF Y. KHAKOO, MD
Assistant Professor, Department of Cardiology, The University of Texas M.D. Anderson Cancer Center, Houston, Texas

ALEXANDER J.F. LAZAR, MD, PhD
Department of Pathology, and Director, Sarcoma Molecular Diagnostics, and Faculty, Sarcoma Research Center, The University of Texas M.D. Anderson Cancer Center, Houston, Texas

BERNADETTE LIEGL, MD
Department of Pathology, Medical University of Graz, Graz, Austria; Department of Pathology, Brigham and Women's Hospital, Harvard Medical School, Boston, Massachusetts

MARTIN PALAVECINO, MD
Postdoctoral Fellow, Department of Surgical Oncology, The University of Texas, M.D. Anderson Cancer Center, Houston, Texas

ALBERTO S. PAPPO, MD
Professor, Department of Pediatrics, Texas Children's Cancer Center, Houston, Texas

SHALIN S. PATEL
Department of Cardiology, The University of Texas M.D. Anderson Cancer Center, Institute of Biosciences and Technology, Houston, Texas

DONALD A. PODOLOFF, MD
Professor, Department of Diagnostic Radiology, The University of Texas M.D. Anderson Cancer Center, Houston, Texas

RICHARD QUEK, MD
Visiting Fellow, Center for Sarcoma and Bone Oncology, Dana-Farber Cancer Institute, Boston, Massachusetts; Department of Medical Oncology, National Cancer Centre Singapore, Singapore, Singapore

MARK ROBSON, MD
Associate Attending Physician, Department of Medicine, Clinical Genetics, Breast Cancer Medicine Services, Memorial Sloan-Kettering Cancer Center, New York, New York

NEETA SOMAIAH, MD
Fellow, Department of Medical Oncology, Fox Chase Cancer Center, Philadelphia, Pennsylvania

MARGARET VON MEHREN, MD
Director of Sarcoma Oncology; and Member, Department of Medical Oncology, Fox Chase Cancer Center, Philadelphia, Pennsylvania

STEPHANE ZALINSKI, MD
Postdoctoral Fellow, Department of Surgical Oncology, The University of Texas, M.D. Anderson Cancer Center, Houston, Texas

Contents

> Gastrointestinal stromal tumors (GIST) are the most common mesenchy-
> mal tumors of the gastrointestinal tract and are a relatively recently identi-
> fied category of mesenchymal tumors. Germline mutations in a number of
> different genes predispose to GIST. This article discusses familial GIST
> syndrome, Carney triad, Carney-Stratakis syndrome, and neurofibromato-
> sis type 1, and addresses the recognition of an inherited predisposition in
> GIST patients.

> Gastrointestinal stromal tumors (GISTs) rarely occur in pediatric patients,
> but increased recognition of adult GIST has led to better awareness of
> the existence of this entity in the pediatric population. GIST occurring in
> pediatric patients has a unique biology and clinical behavior and warrants
> discussion as an independent entity. The generally accepted definition of
> pediatric GIST is a tumor that is diagnosed at the age of 18 years or youn-
> ger. This review highlights the clinical features, molecular biology, and clin-
> ical management of this rare pediatric entity.

> While gastrointestinal stromal tumors have been increasingly recognized
> with the prolonged survival and highly effective new targeted treatments,
> the role of imaging has become important not only for diagnosing and
> staging the tumors, but also for monitoring the effects of treatment and
> surveillance. Computed tomography is the imaging modality of choice
> for these purposes. Fluorine-18 fluorodeoxyglucose positron emission to-
> mography is primarily used in problem solving when there are inconsis-
> tencies between CT and clinical findings or inconclusive CT images. The
> roles of MRI and ultrasound are also described.

> Gastrointestinal stromal tumors (GISTs) are the most common mesenchy-
> mal tumors of the gastrointestinal tract. The vast majority of GISTs harbor
> a *KIT* or *PDGFRA* mutation and express KIT by immunohistochemistry.

However, KIT-negative tumors and tumors showing unusual morphologic features can cause major diagnostic problems. The ability to inhibit the active KIT or PDGFRA kinase with tyrosine kinase inhibitors and alternative drugs demands more than ever accurate tumor classification and risk assessment. This article focuses on the pathology of GIST, including unusual variants and morphologic changes resulting from treatment. Parameters for risk assessment, potentially helpful new immunohistochemical markers, differential diagnosis, and the application of molecular classification schemes are discussed.

Gastrointestinal stromal tumor (GIST) is a disease that was poorly understood historically. In the last decade, it has undergone a major transformation, sparked by the landmark discovery of the central role of activating *KIT* mutations in its pathogenesis and recognition of KIT protein expression (CD 117) as a reliable diagnostic marker of disease. The introduction and subsequent US Food and Drug administration approval of imatinib mesylate in the treatment of metastatic or unresectable GIST in February 1, 2002 has thrust this hitherto little known disease into the center stage of oncology, and GIST has served as a model for rationally designed drug trials in the field of cancer therapeutics since.

Gastrointestinal stromal tumor (GIST) is a rare neoplasm that recently has become an intense focus of scientific investigation, as it serves as a model for the molecular therapy for cancer. Although surgery remains the principle treatment of primary localized GIST, imatinib mesylate, a selective inhibitor of KIT protein, achieves dramatic responses in metastatic GIST. Multimodality therapy integrating surgery and molecular therapy has shown promise. This article summarizes the epidemiology, clinicopathologic features, natural history, and clinical management of GIST.

Small-molecule tyrosine kinase inhibitors (TKIs) have revolutionized the targeted treatment of various cancers, including gastrointestinal stromal tumors (GISTs). Recent evidence suggests the possibility of cardiotoxicity secondary to TKI treatment of GISTs. Preclinical studies indicate that imatinib and sunitinib may be directly toxic to cardiac myocytes. Clinically, cardiotoxicity attributable to imatinib seems to be infrequent and manageable, whereas that attributable to sunitinib is more common and more severe. Further prospective studies with objective cardiac monitoring and long-term follow up are needed to define more accurately the incidence, natural history, and risk factors for developing cardiotoxicity associated with TKIs used in the treatment of patients who have GISTs. In this review, the authors discuss what is known regarding the cardiovascular effects of TKIs used in the treatment of GISTs.

Imatinib mesylate and perifosine are two relatively new drugs that have improved outcomes for patients with gastrointestinal stromal tumors in recent years. The ocular side effects of these two drugs are discussed in this chapter. The most common ocular side effect associated with imatinib mesylate is periorbital edema. Perifosine has been associated with a ring-shaped perilimbal corneal ulceration that can be treated with topical steroids and topical antibiotics.

Liver resection is the preferred treatment for gastrointestinal stromal tumor liver metastases (GIST LMs) when complete resection can be achieved. Major and extended hepatic resections can be safely performed, and using modern techniques, an increasing proportion of patients with GIST LMs are candidates for potentially curative therapy. The combination of tyrosine kinase inhibitor therapy (eg, imatinib) with surgery seems to improve outcome, and although prospective data are lacking, a short neoadjuvant course (6 months) of imatinib therapy followed by resection may improve patient selection for surgery and outcome from treatment. Postoperative therapy with imatinib is generally advised, although the duration of such therapy is not yet clearly defined. These questions may formulate the basis for future prospective studies of imatinib with complete resection of GIST LMs.

Gastrointestinal stromal tumors (GISTs) are the most common mesenchymal neoplasm of the gastrointestinal tract. The interventional radiologist plays an important role in the diagnosis and locoregional therapy for metastatic GISTs. Radiofrequency ablation (RFA) is a potentially curative option for patients exhibiting partial response to imatinib with focal residual disease. RFA can also be used for local control of focal hepatic or peritoneal metastasis. Hepatic embolization or chemoembolization is reserved for the treatment of progressive liver disease in imatinib-resistant patients who are not suitable for sunitinib as a second-line therapy.

The management of advanced gastronintestinal stromal tumor is increasingly complex because of imatinib refractory disease. Primary resistance to imatinib is uncommon, and most patients progress after development of additional genetic changes. This article reviews management strategies including surgical approaches, local modalities for progressive liver metastases, as well as novel therapeutic agents.

RELATED INTEREST
Gastrointestinal Endoscopy Clinics, July 2005 (Vol. 15, No. 3)
Endoscopy and Oncology
M.L. Kochman and J.N. Shah, *Guest Editors*

THE CLINICS ARE NOW AVAILABLE ONLINE!

Access your subscription at:
www.theclinics.com

Preface

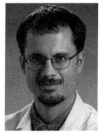 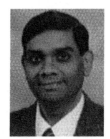

Jonathan C. Trent, MD, PhD   Shreyaskumar R. Patel, MD
Guest Editors

Over the previous 5 decades, basic scientists, pathologists, and clinicians have studied and struggled with gastrointestinal stromal tumors (GISTs) without any major advances in patient care and outcomes. However, over the last decade, discoveries made by these investigators have led to an understanding of the biological role of Kit mutation in GISTs and the development of one of the most exciting examples of targeted therapy to date.

The success of Kit tyrosine kinase inhibitors, such as imatinib mesylate (Gleevec, formerly STI-571) and sunitinib maleate (Sutent), are unprecedented in the therapy of solid tumors. Thus, it is not surprising that the combination of a molecularly-targeted therapy in a molecularly-driven disease has led to several new paradigms in the treatment of cancer, culminating in the concept of personalized therapy for a given individual.

In this issue of *Hematology/Oncology Clinics of North America* we have decided to focus on specific aspects of GIST that set this disease and its therapy apart from other types of cancer. The issue begins with a comprehensive review of the inherited syndromes that predispose an individual to developing GIST, followed by the special situation of pediatric GIST that is hereditary in some circumstances and full of therapeutic unknowns. The article on imaging in GIST illustrates the diagnostic and therapeutic assessments that have led to the development of new response criteria for this disease, which better depict the true efficacy of the agent. The conventional and molecular histopathologic approaches to the diagnosis and risk stratification of primary GIST are in constant evolution as discussed herein. The clinical overview section provides a foundation for truly understanding not only the contemporary clinical approach to the management of GIST, but also the remarkable progress made in the therapy of patients who have this previously rapidly fatal disease. The recent approval of adjuvant imatinib for the treatment of patients who have resected primary GIST sets the stage for the articles on the use of surgery in GIST. Although molecular therapies, such as imatinib and sunitinib, generally are better tolerated than cytotoxic chemotherapy, they do have their own set of side effects, including some unique ones

Hematol Oncol Clin N Am 23 (2009) xiii–xiv
doi:10.1016/j.hoc.2009.01.002
0889-8588/09/$ – see front matter   **hemonc.theclinics.com**

presented in the articles on cardiovascular and ocular effects of these agents in GIST patients. In addition to systemic therapies, patients who have GIST have been found to benefit from local therapy of limited progression after imatinib, such as partial hepatic resection and hepatic arterial embolization. Finally, the issue concludes with an overview of new therapeutic agents currently in clinical trial or in clinical development.

Imatinib quickly has become the most active targeted, small molecule therapy in solid tumors. Imatinib is the first-line agent for metastatic GIST and recently has been approved for the adjuvant therapy of patients who have resected, primary GIST. The marked efficacy of Kit inhibitors in GIST is profound, but so is the number of new questions that each new development elicits. Should patients who have exon 9 mutation in Kit be treated initially with 800mg daily of imatinib? Should patients who have exon 9 mutation or expression of VEGF be treated with sunitinib in front-line? What is the appropriate duration of adjuvant therapy: 1 year, 2 years, 5 years? Should germ-line Kit mutation testing be performed on patients who have a hereditary predisposition syndrome for GIST?

Continued research and clinical investigation is required to answer these questions. The ensuing understanding of disease will lead to additional therapeutic advances and, no doubt, additional unanswered questions.

Jonathan C. Trent, MD, PhD

Shreyaskumar R. Patel, MD
Department of Sarcoma Medical Oncology
The University of Texas M.D. Anderson Cancer Center
1515 Holcombe Boulevard
FC11.3022, Unit 450
Houston, TX 77030, USA

E-mail addresses:
jtrent@mdanderson.org (J.C. Trent)
spatel@mdanderson.org (S.R. Patel)

Inherited Predisposition to Gastrointestinal Stromal Tumor

Rinki Agarwal, MBBS[a], Mark Robson, MD[b],*

KEYWORDS

- Gastrointestinal stromal tumor • Germline • c-KIT
- PDGFRA • Neurofibromatosis • Carney-Stratakis

Gastrointestinal (GI) stromal tumors (GIST) are the most common mesenchymal tumors of the gastrointestinal tract. GIST were first thought to be neoplasms of smooth muscle origin, but Mazur and Clark[1] demonstrated in 1983 that these tumors did not have the ultrastructural characteristics of smooth muscle cells. GIST are now believed to arise from the interstitial cells of Cajal (ICC), the "pacemakers" of the GI tract. In 1998, Hirota and colleagues[2] described gain-of-function mutations in the c-*KIT* proto-oncogene in sporadic GIST tumors. KIT protein expression, identified by CD117 positivity, is present in over 90% of sporadic GIST. Most GIST also express CD34. Somatic activation of c-*KIT* and over-expression of KIT protein are central to the pathogenesis of many GIST tumors, and inhibition of KIT activity by small molecules, such as imatinib and sunitinib, often results in dramatic clinical responses. A small proportion of GIST do not manifest somatic c-*KIT* mutations. Some of these tumors contain mutations in platelet-derived growth factor receptor α (*PDGFRA*). Others, particularly in pediatric GIST, do not have mutations in either of these genes.

EPIDEMIOLOGY

There are few epidemiologic studies of GIST because of the relatively recent recognition of these tumors as an independent entity. The annual incidence in recent publications has ranged from 6.8 to 14.6 per million.[3–9] The peak incidence of GIST tumors appears to be in the seventh decade of life, with an approximately equal gender distribution. GIST are observed in persons of all races. To date, no specific risk factors for

[a] Department of Medicine, Clinical Genetics, Memorial Sloan-Kettering Cancer Center, 1275 York Avenue, New York, NY 10065, USA
[b] Department of Medicine, Clinical Genetics and Breast Cancer Medicine Services, Memorial Sloan-Kettering Cancer Center, 1275 York Avenue, New York, NY 10065, USA
* Corresponding author.
E-mail address: robsonm@mskcc.org (M. Robson).

Hematol Oncol Clin N Am 23 (2009) 1–13
doi:10.1016/j.hoc.2008.12.003
0889-8588/08/$ – see front matter © 2009 Elsevier Inc. All rights reserved.

hemonc.theclinics.com

GIST have been described. The risk of GIST in family members of patients with GIST is not known, although familial aggregations have been described (see below).

INHERITED PREDISPOSITION TO GASTROINTESTINAL STROMAL TUMOR

In 1998, Nishida and colleagues[10] described a Japanese family in which three individuals in two generations were diagnosed with multiple GIST. Several other family members had been described as suffering from symptoms that were consistent with GIST, although these diagnoses were not documented. The proband and her nephew described perineal hyperpigmentation. The germline DNA of the available affected family members contained a germline mutation in exon 11 of c-*KIT*, which resulted in deletion of a valine residue at codon 559_560, the juxta-membrane domain of the KIT protein. This deletion, also observed in the subjects' GIST tumors, was shown to result in constitutive activation of KIT. Families with similar features had been reported as early as 1990,[11] but the report by Nishida and colleagues was the first to identify a specific germline mutation as the cause of an inherited predisposition to GIST. Since that time, it has become clear that GIST can be a manifestation of several different hereditary syndromes.

FAMILIAL GASTROINTESTINAL STROMAL TUMOR SYNDROME

Since the original description by Nishida and colleagues,[12–32] 20 similar families have been described (**Table 1**). Germline mutations of c-*KIT* were identified in 17 of these families,[12,13,16–28,30–32] and mutations in *PDFGRA* in three.[14,15,29] The descriptions of the families are retrospective, and clinical details were not always verified by examination or records review. Thus, it is not entirely clear whether the described clinical heterogeneity reflects variable penetrance of different features, or simply variable reporting. Prospective studies of familial GIST are presently underway to address this uncertainty.

Age and Gender

In the two largest kindreds with familial GIST, the mean age at GIST diagnosis was 49 to 54.[23,30] The median age at diagnosis in all the reported kindreds is 47.5 years, ranging from 18 to 80 years. While the median age at diagnosis appears to be at least a decade younger than typical for sporadic GIST, the precise age at diagnosis is not known for many family members in the families that have been described to date. In one report, there appeared to be a birth cohort effect, with more recent generations being diagnosed younger than older generations.[30] Such an effect was not noted in a second large kindred, however.[23] Males and females appeared to be affected equally.

Gastrointestinal Stromal Tumor Location and Histology

Individuals with familial GIST syndrome (FGS) typically develop multiple GIST, usually located in the small bowel or, less commonly, stomach (**Fig. 1**). Isolated involvement of the stomach histologic appears to be less prevalent than in sporadic GIST. Familial GIST have been described in other locations, such as the esophagus and rectum.[32] Apart from the multiplicity, the histologic appearance of the GIST in FGS appears to be similar to that of sporadic GIST. Most reported cases express KIT protein (CD117) and are also CD34 positive. When described, mitotic rates appear to be low, although metastatic disease has been reported even with tumors that manifest relatively low mitotic rates.[23] Diffuse hyperplasia of the myenteric (Auerbach's) plexus in association with multiple GIST was first described by O'Brien and colleagues[19,27] in

Table 1
Reported familial GIST syndrome kindreds

Gene (Exon)	Mutation	Domain	Kindred	Pigmentation	Urticaria	Nevi	Dysphagia
KIT (8)	del419D	JM	Hartman 2005[17]	ND	+	ND	ND
	W557R	JM	O'Brien 1999[19,27,23]	ND	ND	ND	ND
			Robson 2004[30]	+	No	No	+
	V559del	JM	Nishida 1998[10]	+	ND	ND	ND
KIT (11)	V559A	JM	Beghini 2001[12]	+	+	ND	ND
			Maeyama 2001[26]	+	No	ND	ND
			Kim 2005[22]	No	No	No	No
			Li 2005[25]	+	+	+	ND
	Ins576QL577	—	Kang 2007[21]	ND	ND	ND	ND
	Q575_P577delinsH	JM	Carballo 2005[13]	+	ND	No	No
	D579del	JM	Woznaik 2008[32]	No	No	ND	ND
		TK1	Tarn 2005[31]	ND	ND	ND	ND
		—	Lasota 2006[24]	ND	ND	ND	ND
		—	Kleinbaum 2008[23]	ND	ND	ND	ND
KIT (13)	K642E	TK1	Isozaki 2000[20]	No	ND	ND	ND
			Graham 2007[16]	No	No	No	No
KIT (17)	D820Y	TK2	Hirota 2002[18]	ND	ND	ND	+
			O'Riain 2005[28]	ND	ND	ND	+
PDGFRA[a]	Y555C	—	De Raedt 2006[15]	ND	ND	ND	ND
	V561D	—	Pasini 2007[29]	ND	ND	ND	ND
	D846Y	—	Chompret 2004[14]	No	No	No	No

Abbreviation: ND, Not described (usually not specifically mentioned as present as present or absent).
[a] PDGFRA kindreds reported as having "large hands."

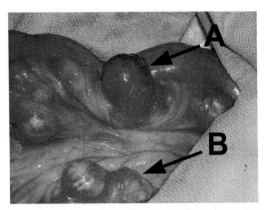

Fig. 1. Gross appearance of small bowel in FGS. (A) and (B) indicate GIST tumors.

1999 in a family that was subsequently shown to be transmitting a c-*KIT* mutation. This finding has since been described in many kindreds with FGS and c-*KIT* mutations, and likely reflects polyclonal activation of the ICC by the mutated protein.[33] Additional mutation events (such as deletions of chromosomes 14 and 22) are probably necessary to transform the target cells into clinically evident GIST.[25] The clinical behavior of the GIST tumors in FGS has varied in different reports. In the experience of Robson and colleagues, death from metastatic GIST was not documented while, in the large series of Kleinbaum and colleagues, 9 of 11 patients not treated with imatinib died of metastatic GIST.[23,30] The factors responsible for the variation in clinical outcome have not been clarified.

Associated Clinical Findings

Members of FGS kindreds may manifest cutaneous findings, such as hyperpigmentation, urticaria pigmentosa, or increased numbers of nevi. The hyperpigmentation is most commonly perineal in distribution, although changes may also be noted on the hands, elbows, knees, and face (**Fig. 2**). In one family, the changes were described as being more prominent in childhood, with a tendency to fade with age. In the affected areas, the pigmentation is often more diffuse than speckled, although families with multiple nevi and lentigines have also been described.[25] Mast cell disease has been described in some families, manifesting as urticaria pigmentosa or even systemic mastocytosis.

Dysphagia has been described by members of several FGS families. In the family described by Marshall and colleagues,[11] this was thought to be related to "esophageal leiomyomatosis" and achlasia. Although the clinical description of this family is consistent with FGS, no germline abnormality has been reported in this particular kindred. In other FGS families with dysphagia, physical obstruction by esophageal GIST has not been common. The physiology of dysphagia appears to be different from that in true achalasia, although manometric findings were abnormal in one report.[18] In that family, several members demonstrated circular thickening of the distal esophageal wall with simultaneous and repetitive low-amplitude esophageal contraction. Additional studies may more completely delineate the etiology of FGS-associated dysphagia.

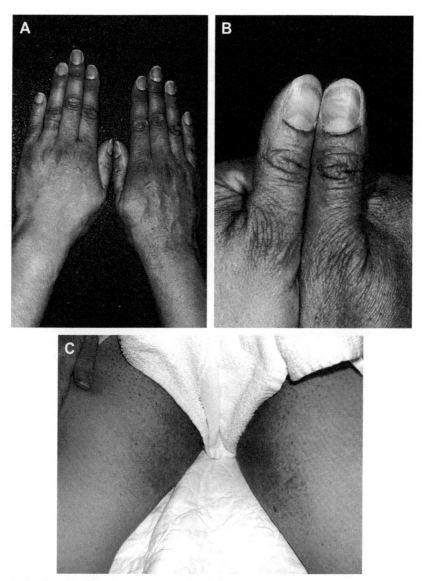

Fig. 2. (*A–C*) Perineal and hand pigmentation in FGS.

Genetics

In the FGS kindreds studied to date, the most common germline abnormality has been a germline mutation in c-*KIT*, typically resulting in alteration of the juxta-membrane domain (See **Table 1**). Mutations have also been reported in both tyrosine kinase domains, however. Most mutations have been observed in exon 11, although exons 8, 13, and 17 mutations have also been described. All c-*KIT* mutations associated with FGS are believed to constitutively active the KIT protein. Three families with FGS have been reported in which the germline abnormality was a mutation in the *PDGRFA* gene.

Although all c-*KIT* and *PDGFRA* mutations appear to predispose to GIST, no differences have been reported with respect to age of onset, site of GIST, or clinical course in families with different mutations. The available clinical reports suggest that there may be a correlation between the site of mutation and associated clinical features. All three major manifestations (GIST, cutaneous findings, dysphagia) have been observed in kindreds with exon 11 mutations, but pigmented lesions were not described in kindreds with exon 13 and 17 mutations. Systemic mastocytosis was observed with GIST in a family with a mutation in exon 8 of c-*KIT* (D419del), and a germline exon 9 mutation (K509I) has been described presenting with familial systemic mastocytosis, but without GIST.[34] The presence of dysphagia is not clearly linked to mutations in any specific region. Cutaneous findings and dysphagia have not been described in families with mutations in *PDGFRA*, but "unusually large hands" were reported in these families.[14,15] Taken together, these reports suggest that there may be variation in clinical presentation according the gene mutated and the site of mutation. However, phenotypes have not been routinely verified by complete physical examination, and thus features may be present but not noted. In addition, there may be considerable variation in expression of the different features, even within a family. For example, in one large kindred, hyperpigmentation was only described in five of eight (62.5%) documented mutation carriers.[30] The absence of a feature in a specific individual does not, therefore, preclude an association with the mutation observed in that individual.

Inheritance Pattern and Penetrance

FGS appears to be an autosomal dominant syndrome, with no gender predilection. The penetrance appears to be high, with 15 of 22 documented or obligate carriers being affected by GIST in one large kindred.[30] The risk of clinically diagnosed GIST appears to be 91% to 100% by age 70.[23,30] As mentioned previously, one family appeared to demonstrate a birth cohort effect, with the younger generation being diagnosed at an earlier average age. This effect may have resulted from the development of noninvasive intra-abdominal imaging rather than from genetic anticipation or environmental modulation of penetrance. Another large kindred did not manifest this effect.[23]

Animal Models

The central importance of c-*KIT* in the pathogenesis of GIST has been demonstrated in animal models.[35] Several investigators have described "knock-in" mice that mimic the situation in families transmitting germline c-*KIT* mutations. Sommers and colleagues[36] reported mice with the gain-of-function KIT mutation V558del (corresponding to the human V559del). Heterozygous mice manifested cecal GIST-like tumors and lesions resembling diffuse ICC hyperplasia distributed through the esophagus, stomach, duodenum, and large intestine. Similar findings were noted in mice homozygous for KIT K641Q (analogous to human K642Q) and either heterozygous or homozygous for KIT D818Y (analogous to the human exon 17 mutation D820Y).[37,38] Perhaps surprisingly, KIT D818Y mice did not demonstrate ICC hyperplasia in the small intestine, the most common site of human tumors in FGS. Abnormalities in lower esophageal pigmentation were variably present in the different models (present in V558del and D818Y but not in K641Q). Increased dermal mast cells were only noted in the mice with V558del, the exon 11 mutation. These findings suggest that KIT activation from whatever mechanism produces ICC hyperplasia and GIST, but different mutations have differing effects in stimulation of melanocytes and mast cells.

CARNEY TRIAD AND CARNEY-STRATAKIS SYNDROME

Gastric GIST are components of two eponymous and easily confused syndromes, Carney triad (CT) and Carney-Stratakis syndrome (CSS). CT was first described in 1977 when Carney and colleagues[39] reported seven unrelated women who presented with combinations of gastric epithelioid leiomyosarcomas (now thought to be GIST), pulmonary chondromas, and extra-adrenal paragangliomas. Subsequently, Carney described a series of 79 patients with at least two of these three component tumors.[40] Although a few cases have been described since then, there are fewer than 100 cases in the world literature. Most (85%) cases have occurred in woman, and most (82%) were diagnosed before age 30. A family history of a component tumor was rare, and CT is thought to be a sporadic condition. Individuals with family histories of GIST or paraganglioma are more likely to have CSS (see below). Transmission of CT to offspring has not been documented and no germline mutation has been identified.

In his 1999 review of CT, Carney reported that most patients presented with gastric GIST, and a substantial number had metastatic disease at presentation or developed it during follow-up.[40] Even in the absence of systemic metastasis, metachronous gastric disease was commonly diagnosed after subtotal gastrectomy at a median of 12 years of follow-up. In contrast to sporadic GIST, tumors associated with CT appear not to over-express KIT protein and do not contain somatic mutations in c-KIT or PDGFRA.[41,42] comparative genomic hybridization (CGH) analysis rarely demonstrates the 14q and 22q losses that are frequently seen in sporadic GIST. The most common CGH anomaly appears to be loss on 1q, although several tumors demonstrated no losses at all by CGH.[43]

Although the majority of patients with CT have no family members with any of the triad component tumors, Carney noted in his 1999 review that two patients had siblings with a component tumor, raising the possibility that a subset of CT could be familial. In 2002, Carney and Stratakis described these two families and three others in which there was an apparent familial predisposition.[44] Of the 12 patients, 7 had paraganglioma, 4 had paraganglioma and gastric GIST, and 1 had gastric GIST alone. As with CT, patients were initially diagnosed at an early age (mean 23), but both males and females were affected and there were no pulmonary chondromas. The investigators coined the term "Carney-Stratakis Syndrome" to describe patients and families with the paraganglioma/gastric GIST dyad.

CSS appears to be an autosomal dominant predisposition syndrome, with incomplete penetrance and variable manifestation. In particular, susceptible individuals may develop paraganglioma, GIST, or both. In one report of monozygotic twins with CSS, one twin developed a paraganglioma and the other GIST.[45] Recently, mutations in the SDHB, SDHC, and SDHD succinate dehydrogenase subunits have been described in CSS kindreds.[46] In the largest series to date (11 individuals from 9 families), mutations were identified in seven kindreds.[47] Notably, mutations were not identified in two families, one of which contained two siblings with multiple paragangliomas, one of whom had GIST. The other mutation-negative family contained three siblings with paragangliomas, one of whom also had GIST. These families suggest either limited sensitivity of testing for mutations in the associated genes, or the presence of additional genes that may be mutated in the syndrome.

NEUROFIBROMATOSIS TYPE 1

Neurofibromatosis type 1 (NF1; von Reckinghausen's Disease) is a complex disorder with a highly variable phenotype, occurring in up to 1 in every 3,000 live births. The most characteristic findings are cutaneous (café au lait spots, axillary and inguinal freckling, multiple dermal neurofibromas) and ocular (hamartomas in the iris called Lisch nodules).[48] Numerous other manifestations have been described, including bony complications and various nervous system tumors, including gliomas (especially optic) and malignant peripheral nerve sheath tumors. NF1 results from germline mutations in the gene encoding the GTPase activating protein neurofibromin, and is inherited in an autosomal dominant manner. Approximately half of the cases, however, occur in the absence of a family history of NF1 and are presumably the result of de novo mutation.

NF1 has several gastrointestinal manifestations, and both myenteric plexus hyperplasia and GIST have been described.[49] The clinical features of NF1-associated GIST resemble those of FGS more than of CT and CSS.[50,51] Tumors tend to be diagnosed in patients who are in their late fifth or sixth decade of life, with a slight female predominance. The NF1 GIST are most often small, multiple, and most commonly distributed in the small bowel. Histologically, the tumors usually have low mitotic rates. Skenioid fibers can be identified with appreciable frequency. KIT protein expression is highly prevalent. S100 expression may be noted in a subset of NF1 GIST, which may give rise to confusion as to whether these tumors represent nerve sheath tumors. Although some reports have observed c-*KIT* or *PDGFRA* mutations in a small proportion of NF1 GIST,[51] other investigators have not confirmed this finding.[50,52] This suggests that NF1 GIST may arise through a non-KIT mediated pathway, or that KIT is activated indirectly by the neurofibromin mutation. If the KIT expression is an epiphenomenon, imatinib and other KIT inhibitors may be of limited utility. The clinical experience with these agents in NF1 GIST is limited, although one case report did suggest disease stabilization with sunitinib treatment.[53]

RECOGNITION AND MANAGEMENT OF INHERITED PREDISPOSITION TO GASTROINTESTINAL STROMAL TUMOR

GIST can be a component of a number of clinical distinct syndromes (**Table 2**). The proportion of GIST that can be attributed to a germline predisposition is currently not known. A multicenter study has recently opened to address this question (details available at https://projectflag.org). Those caring for patients with GIST should consider the possibility of an underlying germline mutation in certain clinical situations. Multicentric disease is suggestive, particularly when present in the small bowel and in younger patients. Careful skin examination may reveal abnormal pigmentation suggestive of FGS or NF1 (hyperpigmentation, urticaria pigmentosa, cafe au lait spots, dermal neurofibromas). A careful family history may reveal other family members who have manifested GIST, NF1, or paragangliomas (which would be suggestive of CSS). Although GIST are not clearly associated with the Li-Fraumeni syndrome (caused by germline p53 mutations), a family history of gastric or intra-abdominal sarcoma (especially leiomyosarcoma) should raise the possibility that the family member may also have had GIST, and that FGS or one of the other syndromes may be present. Pulmonary radiographic findings in young women with gastric GIST should raise the question of possible pulmonary chondromas as part of Carney triad.

There is no evidence that GIST arising as the result of an inherited predisposition should necessarily be treated differently than nonhereditary GIST, or that the presence of a hereditary predisposition constitutes an independent prognostic factor. Indeed, many GIST arising in this setting appear to have favorable histologic features, and prolonged survival has been described, even in the setting of multiple unresected GIST. Surgical resection should be performed when technically feasible and clinically

Table 2
Syndromes associated with predisposition to GIST

Syndrome	Sporadic	Familial GIST	Carney Triad	Carney-Stratakis Syndrome	NF1
Average age at GIST	Approximately 60 years	Approximately 40–50 years	<35 years	<25 years	Approximately 50 years
Gender predilection	None	None	F > M	None	None
Multicentric disease	Rare	Yes	±	Yes	—
Associated features	None	Pigmentation, urticaria pigmentosa, mastocytosis, dysphagia	Paraganglioma, pulmonary chondroma	Paraganglioma	Neuro-fibromas, café au lait spots
Mutations	None (germline)	kit/PDGFRA	Unknown	SDHB SDHC SDHD	Neurofibromin
Inheritance	—	Autosomal dominant	—	Autosomal dominant	Autosomal dominant
Histology	Spindled > epithelioid > mixed	Similar to sporadic	Epithelioid	Similar to sporadic	Spindled cell
ICC hyperplasia	None	Usually present	None	None	Usually present
Location	Stomach, small intestine, rectum, mesentery, gall bladder, other sites	Stomach, small intestine, rarely rectum	Stomach	Stomach	Small intestine
Clinical behavior	Depends on tumor size, site, mitoses	Similar to sporadic GISTs	Significant number have metastases at presentation	Unknown	Indolent
Response to imatinib	Depends on mutation type	Depends on mutation type	Unknown	Poor	Unknown

appropriate. Imatinib or sunitinib therapy should be offered for standard clinical indications, as both FGS and NF1 GIST have been reported to respond. Whether CT/CSS GIST, which do not over-express KIT, will respond is less clear.

If a germline mutation can be identified in a patient with a suspected predisposition to GIST, presymptomatic genetic testing may be considered for unaffected family members. Those who are found not to share the mutation can be reassured that their risk for GIST is likely no greater than that of the general population, which may provide an immense psychologic benefit. Management of those who are shown to share the predisposition may be more challenging, as there is no robust evidence base upon which to ground recommendations. Several investigators have recommended periodic imaging with computed tomography or positron emission tomography. However, it is not clear whether surgical intervention would necessarily be warranted in the absence of clinical symptoms such as pain, bleeding, or obstruction. While it is attractive to consider the preventive use of imatinib or sunitinib in this situation, especially for FGS, the benefits of this approach have not been defined and the risks of lifelong exposure to these agents are not known. "Chemoprevention" of hereditary GIST must therefore be considered an investigational intervention. Finally, individuals of childbearing age who carry the responsible mutation may wish to use that information to guide reproductive decision-making, particularly with regards to the possibility of preimplantation genetic diagnosis.[54]

SUMMARY

Gastrointestinal stromal tumors are a relatively recently identified category of mesenchymal tumors. Germline mutations in a number of different genes predispose to GIST. These "experiments of nature" may provide useful insights into the pathogenesis of the disease. Recognition of an inherited predisposition in a GIST patient does not yet appear to have major impact upon that person's treatment, but the information may nonetheless be useful for presymptomatic family members wishing to delineate their own risk.

REFERENCES

1. Mazur MT, Clark HB. Gastric stromal tumors. Reappraisal of histogenesis. Am J Surg Pathol 1983;7(6):507–19.
2. Hirota S, Isozaki K, Moriyama Y, et al. Gain-of-function mutations of c-kit in human gastrointestinal stromal tumors. Science 1998;279(5350):577–80.
3. Bumming P, Ahlman H, Andersson J, et al. Population-based study of the diagnosis and treatment of gastrointestinal stromal tumours. Br J Surg 2006;93(7): 836–43.
4. Goettsch WG, Bos SD, Breekveldt-Postma N, et al. Incidence of gastrointestinal stromal tumours is underestimated: results of a nation-wide study. Eur J Cancer 2005;41(18):2868–72.
5. Mucciarini C, Rossi G, Bertolini F, et al. Incidence and clinicopathologic features of gastrointestinal stromal tumors. A population-based study. BMC Cancer 2007; 7:230.
6. Nilsson B, Bumming P, Meis-Kindblom JM, et al. Gastrointestinal stromal tumors: the incidence, prevalence, clinical course, and prognostication in the preimatinib mesylate era—a population-based study in western Sweden. Cancer 2005; 103(4):821–9.

7. Perez EA, Livingstone AS, Franceschi D, et al. Current incidence and outcomes of gastrointestinal mesenchymal tumors including gastrointestinal stromal tumors. J Am Coll Surg 2006;202(4):623–9.

8. Rubio J, Marcos-Gragera R, Ortiz MR, et al. Population-based incidence and survival of gastrointestinal stromal tumours (GIST) in Girona, Spain. Eur J Cancer 2007;43(1):144–8.

9. Tran T, Davila JA, El-Serag HB. The epidemiology of malignant gastrointestinal stromal tumors: an analysis of 1,458 cases from 1992 to 2000. Am J Gastroenterol 2005;100(1):162–8.

10. Nishida T, Hirota S, Taniguchi M, et al. Familial gastrointestinal stromal tumours with germline mutation of the KIT gene. Nat Genet 1998;19(4):323–4.

11. Marshall JB, Diaz-Arias AA, Bochna GS, et al. Achalasia due to diffuse esophageal leiomyomatosis and inherited as an autosomal dominant disorder. Report of a family study. Gastroenterology 1990;98(5 Pt 1):1358–65.

12. Beghini A, Tibiletti MG, Roversi G, et al. Germline mutation in the juxtamembrane domain of the kit gene in a family with gastrointestinal stromal tumors and urticaria pigmentosa. Cancer 2001;92(3):657–62.

13. Carballo M, Roig I, Aguilar F, et al. Novel c-KIT germline mutation in a family with gastrointestinal stromal tumors and cutaneous hyperpigmentation. Am J Med Genet A 2005;132(4):361–4.

14. Chompret A, Kannengiesser C, Barrois M, et al. PDGFRA germline mutation in a family with multiple cases of gastrointestinal stromal tumor. Gastroenterology 2004;126(1):318–21.

15. de Raedt T, Cools J, Debiec-Rychter M, et al. Intestinal neurofibromatosis is a subtype of familial GIST and results from a dominant activating mutation in PDGFRA. Gastroenterology 2006;131(6):1907–12.

16. Graham J, Debiec-Rychter M, Corless CL, et al. Imatinib in the management of multiple gastrointestinal stromal tumors associated with a germline KIT K642E mutation. Arch Pathol Lab Med 2007;131(9):1393–6.

17. Hartmann K, Wardelmann E, Ma Y, et al. Novel germline mutation of KIT associated with familial gastrointestinal stromal tumors and mastocytosis. Gastroenterology 2005;129(3):1042–6.

18. Hirota S, Nishida T, Isozaki K, et al. Familial gastrointestinal stromal tumors associated with dysphagia and novel type germline mutation of KIT gene. Gastroenterology 2002;122(5):1493–9.

19. Hirota S, Okazaki T, Kitamura Y, et al. Cause of familial and multiple gastrointestinal autonomic nerve tumors with hyperplasia of interstitial cells of Cajal is germline mutation of the c-kit gene. Am J Surg Pathol 2000;24(2):326–7.

20. Isozaki K, Terris B, Belghiti J, et al. Germline-activating mutation in the kinase domain of KIT gene in familial gastrointestinal stromal tumors. Am J Pathol 2000;157(5):1581–5.

21. Kang DY, Park CK, Choi JS, et al. Multiple gastrointestinal stromal tumors: clinicopathologic and genetic analysis of 12 patients. Am J Surg Pathol 2007;31(2):224–32.

22. Kim HJ, Lim SJ, Park K, et al. Multiple gastrointestinal stromal tumors with a germline c-kit mutation. Pathol Int 2005;55(10):655–9.

23. Kleinbaum EP, Lazar AJ, Tamborini E, et al. Clinical, histopathologic, molecular and therapeutic findings in a large kindred with gastrointestinal stromal tumor. Int J Cancer 2008;122(3):711–8.

24. Lasota J, Miettinen M. A new familial GIST identified. Am J Surg Pathol 2006;30(10):1342.

25. Li FP, Fletcher JA, Heinrich MC, et al. Familial gastrointestinal stromal tumor syndrome: phenotypic and molecular features in a kindred. J Clin Oncol 2005; 23(12):2735–43.
26. Maeyama H, Hidaka E, Ota H, et al. Familial gastrointestinal stromal tumor with hyperpigmentation: association with a germline mutation of the c-kit gene. Gastroenterology 2001;120(1):210–5.
27. O'Brien P, Kapusta L, Dardick I, et al. Multiple familial gastrointestinal autonomic nerve tumors and small intestinal neuronal dysplasia. Am J Surg Pathol 1999; 23(2):198–204.
28. O'Riain C, Corless CL, Heinrich MC, et al. Gastrointestinal stromal tumors: insights from a new familial GIST kindred with unusual genetic and pathologic features. Am J Surg Pathol 2005;29(12):1680–3.
29. Pasini B, Matyakhina L, Bei T, et al. Multiple gastrointestinal stromal and other tumors caused by platelet-derived growth factor receptor alpha gene mutations: a case associated with a germline V561D defect. J Clin Endocrinol Metab 2007; 92(9):3728–32.
30. Robson ME, Glogowski E, Sommer G, et al. Pleomorphic characteristics of a germ-line KIT mutation in a large kindred with gastrointestinal stromal tumors, hyperpigmentation, and dysphagia. Clin Cancer Res 2004;10(4):1250–4.
31. Tarn C, Merkel E, Canutescu AA, et al. Analysis of KIT mutations in sporadic and familial gastrointestinal stromal tumors: therapeutic implications through protein modeling. Clin Cancer Res 2005;11(10):3668–77.
32. Wozniak A, Rutkowski P, Sciot R, et al. Rectal gastrointestinal stromal tumors associated with a novel germline KIT mutation. Int J Cancer 2008;122(9): 2160–4.
33. Chen H, Hirota S, Isozaki K, et al. Polyclonal nature of diffuse proliferation of interstitial cells of Cajal in patients with familial and multiple gastrointestinal stromal tumours. Gut 2002;51(6):793–6.
34. Zhang LY, Smith ML, Schultheis B, et al. A novel K509I mutation of KIT identified in familial mastocytosis-in vitro and in vivo responsiveness to imatinib therapy. Leuk Res 2006;30(4):373–8.
35. Gunawan B. Knock-in murine models of familial gastrointestinal stromal tumours. J Pathol 2008;214(4):407–9.
36. Sommer G, Agosti V, Ehlers I, et al. Gastrointestinal stromal tumors in a mouse model by targeted mutation of the Kit receptor tyrosine kinase. Proc Natl Acad Sci USA 2003;100(11):6706–11.
37. Nakai N, Ishikawa T, Nishitani A, et al. A mouse model of a human multiple GIST family with KIT-Asp820Tyr mutation generated by a knock-in strategy. J Pathol 2008;214(3):302–11.
38. Rubin BP, Antonescu CR, Scott-Browne JP, et al. A knock-in mouse model of gastrointestinal stromal tumor harboring kit K641E. Cancer Res 2005;65(15): 6631–9.
39. Carney JA, Sheps SG, Go VL, et al. The triad of gastric leiomyosarcoma, functioning extra-adrenal paraganglioma and pulmonary chondroma. N Engl J Med 1977;296(26):1517–8.
40. Carney JA. Gastric stromal sarcoma, pulmonary chondroma, and extra-adrenal paraganglioma (Carney Triad): natural history, adrenocortical component, and possible familial occurrence. Mayo Clin Proc 1999;74(6):543–52.
41. Agaimy A, Pelz AF, Corless CL, et al. Epithelioid gastric stromal tumours of the antrum in young females with the Carney triad: a report of three new cases

with mutational analysis and comparative genomic hybridization. Oncol Rep 2007;18(1):9–15.

42. Knop S, Schupp M, Wardelmann E, et al. A new case of Carney triad: gastrointestinal stromal tumours and leiomyoma of the oesophagus do not show activating mutations of KIT and platelet-derived growth factor receptor alpha. J Clin Pathol 2006;59(10):1097–9.

43. Matyakhina L, Bei TA, McWhinney SR, et al. Genetics of Carney triad: recurrent losses at chromosome 1 but lack of germline mutations in genes associated with paragangliomas and gastrointestinal stromal tumors. J Clin Endocrinol Metab 2007;92(8):2938–43.

44. Carney JA, Stratakis CA. Familial paraganglioma and gastric stromal sarcoma: a new syndrome distinct from the Carney triad. Am J Med Genet 2002;108(2): 132–9.

45. Boccon-Gibod L, Boman F, Boudjemaa S, et al. Separate occurrence of extra-adrenal paraganglioma and gastrointestinal stromal tumor in monozygotic twins: probable familial Carney syndrome. Pediatr Dev Pathol 2004;7(4):380–4.

46. McWhinney SR, Pasini B, Stratakis CA. Familial gastrointestinal stromal tumors and germ-line mutations. N Engl J Med 2007;357(10):1054–6.

47. Pasini B, McWhinney SR, Bei T, et al. Clinical and molecular genetics of patients with the Carney-Stratakis syndrome and germline mutations of the genes coding for the succinate dehydrogenase subunits SDHB, SDHC, and SDHD. Eur J Hum Genet 2008;16(1):79–88.

48. Gutmann DH, Aylsworth A, Carey JC, et al. The diagnostic evaluation and multi-disciplinary management of neurofibromatosis 1 and neurofibromatosis 2. JAMA 1997;278(1):51–7.

49. Fuller CE, Williams GT. Gastrointestinal manifestations of type 1 neurofibromatosis (von Recklinghausen's disease). Histopathology 1991;19(1):1–11.

50. Miettinen M, Fetsch JF, Sobin LH, et al. Gastrointestinal stromal tumors in patients with neurofibromatosis 1: a clinicopathologic and molecular genetic study of 45 cases. Am J Surg Pathol 2006;30(1):90–6.

51. Takazawa Y, Sakurai S, Sakuma Y, et al. Gastrointestinal stromal tumors of neurofibromatosis type I (von Recklinghausen's disease). Am J Surg Pathol 2005;29(6): 755–63.

52. Kinoshita K, Hirota S, Isozaki K, et al. Absence of c-kit gene mutations in gastrointestinal stromal tumours from neurofibromatosis type 1 patients. J Pathol 2004; 202(1):80–5.

53. Kalender ME, Sevinc A, Tutar E, et al. Effect of sunitinib on metastatic gastrointestinal stromal tumor in patients with neurofibromatosis type 1: a case report. World J Gastroenterol 2007;13(18):2629–32.

54. Offit K, Sagi M, Hurley K. Preimplantation genetic diagnosis for cancer syndromes: a new challenge for preventive medicine. JAMA 2006;296(22): 2727–30.

Pediatric Gastrointestinal Stromal Tumors

Alberto S. Pappo, MD[a],*, Katherine A. Janeway, MD[b,c]

KEYWORDS

- Pediatric • Gastrointestinal stromal tumors • IGF-1 • Imatinib
- Sunitinib • Carney triad

Gastrointestinal stromal tumors (GISTs) are the most common mesenchymal neoplasms of the gastrointestinal tract in adults.[1] These tumors are presumed to arise from the interstitial cells of Cajal and are characterized by the presence of activating mutations of the KIT or platelet derived growth factor receptor alpha (PDGFRA) proto-oncogenes.[1] The exact incidence of adult GIST is not known, but it is estimated that there are between 4000 and 5000 new cases in the United States annually. This figure reflects the results of population-based studies conducted in Sweden, Iceland, and the United States where the reported annual incidence for this tumor is 14.5, 11, and 6.8 cases per million population, respectively.[2–4] The median age at diagnosis is 60 years, and these tumors most frequently arise in the stomach (50%) and small bowel (25%).[5] Pathologically, 70% of adult GISTs are characterized by a spindle cell histologic subtype and 20% by an epithelioid architecture.[6] In adults, the determinants of malignant potential and clinical behavior include the stage at initial diagnosis, tumor size, mitotic rate, and anatomic location.[6] Activating mutations of KIT or PDGFRA are detected in over 90% of GISTs occurring in adult patients, and the majority of these patients respond to tyrosine kinase inhibitor therapy such as imatinib or sunitinib.[1,7,8]

GISTs rarely occur in pediatric patients, but increased recognition of adult GIST has led to better awareness of the existence of this entity in the pediatric population. GIST occurring in pediatric patients has a unique biology and clinical behavior and warrants discussion as an independent entity. The generally accepted definition of pediatric GIST is a tumor that is diagnosed at the age of 18 years or younger. This review highlights the clinical features, molecular biology, and clinical management of this rare pediatric entity.

[a] Department of Pediatrics, Texas Children's Cancer Center, 6621 Fannin Street, CC1510.00, Houston, TX 77030, USA
[b] Department of Pediatrics, Harvard Medical School, Boston, MA 02115, USA
[c] Dana Farber Cancer Institute, Children's Hospital, 44 Binney Street, Dana 3, Boston, MA 02115, USA
* Corresponding author.
E-mail address: aspappo@txccc.org (A.S. Pappo).

Hematol Oncol Clin N Am 23 (2009) 15–34
doi:10.1016/j.hoc.2008.11.005
0889-8588/08/$ – see front matter

EPIDEMIOLOGY

The incidence of pediatric GIST in the United States is unknown, most likely owing to the relative rarity of the disease, the lack of consensus on how to code these tumors, the difficulties in separating malignant from benign tumors, and the diagnostic confusion that exists with other pathologic entities such as leiomyosarcoma, leiomyoma, or leiomyoblastoma.[9] A small number of series have estimated that pediatric GIST accounts for approximately 2.5% of all pediatric non-rhabdomyosarcomatous soft tissue sarcomas[10] or for 1.4% to 2.6% of all GISTs seen at large centers.[11,12] The Surveillance, Epidemiology and End Results (SEER) section of the National Cancer Institute data for GIST from 2001 to 2005 is depicted in **Table 1** and demonstrates that only 12 "true" cases of pediatric GIST were available for reporting during this period. Clearly, this figure underestimates the actual number of pediatric GISTs, and improved coding mechanisms and increased recognition of this entity are urgently needed to better define the incidence of this rare pediatric tumor.

ASSOCIATED CANCER PREDISPOSITION SYNDROMES

GIST can arise within the context of four well-defined tumor predisposition syndromes which need to be assessed at the time of initial evaluation of a pediatric patient with suspected GIST.

Table 1
Number of cases of gastrointestinal sarcoma reported to the SEER database, 2001–2005

SEER 17 Areas (Age, y)	Study Period					
	2001	2002	2003	2004	2005	2001–2005
00	0	0	0	0	0	0
01–04	0	0	0	0	0	0
05–09	0	0	1	0	0	1
10–14	1	2	0	2	0	5
15–19	1	2	1	1	1	6
20–24	3	1	0	2	1	7
25–29	2	9	4	7	4	26
30–34	7	14	6	5	6	38
35–39	15	15	20	15	16	81
40–44	21	29	23	25	27	125
45–49	34	37	30	33	45	179
50–54	29	57	39	51	42	218
55–59	27	58	62	62	63	272
60–64	43	45	53	51	49	241
65–69	48	66	62	53	46	275
70–74	61	55	65	67	55	303
75–79	48	59	56	52	36	251
80–84	30	39	44	37	36	186
85+	19	22	27	25	31	124
Total	389	510	493	488	458	2338

Carney Triad

In 1977, Carney reported the association of GIST, pulmonary chondroma, and functioning extra-adrenal paraganglioma.[13] Careful follow-up of these patients has revealed that they are at risk for other tumors as well, such as adrenocortical adenomas.[13] Most patients with the Carney triad are females (85%), and the mean age at presentation is 20.2 years; 82% present with clinical manifestations of this syndrome by age 30 years. Over half of the patients present with GIST and pulmonary chondroma, whereas 1% of patients present with pulmonary chondromas and paragangliomas without GIST.[13] GISTs in patients with the Carney triad tend to be multifocal and to arise in the stomach, particularly in the antrum and lesser curvature. Clinical presentation is often anemia due to gastrointestinal bleeding. Local recurrence (46%) and metastasis (55%) to the liver, lymph nodes, and peritoneum are not uncommon, but patients often have an indolent clinical course with recurrences reported as late as 39 years after initial surgery.[13] The Carney triad is sporadic; the underlying defect is not known, and GISTs in these patients lack KIT, PDGFRA, and succinate dehydrogenase (SDH) mutations.[14]

Carney-Stratakis Syndrome

Described in 2002, this syndrome is characterized by the presence of paragangliomas and GIST that are inherited in an autosomal dominant manner with incomplete penetrance.[15] The median age at presentation for these patients is 19 years,[16] and some patients can present with GIST, anemia, and gastrointestinal bleeding in the absence of a coexisting paraganglioma.[15,16] GISTs in these patients more commonly have an intramural and stomach location, exhibit spindle cell morphology, and are multifocal. KIT and PDGFRA mutations are absent,[16] but germline mutations or deletions in the genes for SDH B, C, or D are present in the majority of patients with the Carney-Stratakis syndrome as discussed later.[16,17] These patients also can have adrenocortical adenomas.

Familial Gastrointestinal Stromal Tumors

Germline mutations in KIT or PDGFRA have been reported in 14 families. The median age of diagnosis in patients with familial GIST is 46 years; therefore, this syndrome is less likely to be present in the pediatric population. Nevertheless, it is important to evaluate patients for signs and symptoms associated with KIT and PDGFRA germline mutations which include melanoma, lentigines, urticaria pigmentosa, perioral and perineal hyperpigmentation, and achalasia.[6,18]

Neurofibromatosis Type 1

The association between neurofibromatosis type 1 (NF-1) and GIST is discussed further in the review by Robson elsewhere in this issue. As is true for familial GIST, the median age of GIST diagnosis in NF-1 patients is younger than that observed in adult sporadic GIST (49 years) but outside the pediatric GIST age range.[6] Nevertheless, pediatric patients with GIST should be assessed for the presence of signs and symptoms of NF-1.

CLINICOPATHOLOGIC FEATURES OF PEDIATRIC GASTROINTESTINAL STROMAL TUMORS

The clinical characteristics, molecular findings, and pathologic features of 121 patients with pediatric GIST reported in 28 series or individual case reports are depicted in **Table 2**. The most common manifestations at the time of initial presentation included anemia or symptoms related to it, gastrointestinal bleeding, a palpable abdominal mass, abdominal distension, and intestinal obstruction, particularly in the newborn

Table 2
Clinical, pathologic, and molecular features of 121 pediatric patients with GIST reported in the literature

Study	Number of Patients, Age (y), Sex (F/M)	Location	Pathologic Subtype/Mitosis	Other Relevant Information	KIT/PDFGR Mutations	Imatinib or Sunitinib/ Evaluable Response	Outcome/Comments
Miettinen[11,a]	34 5–18 (median, 13) 27/7	Stomach (n = 34)[a]	Epithelioid (n = 21) Spindle/epithelioid (n = 5) Spindle (n = 8) 0–65/50 (median, 6/50 HPF)	Size 1.5–24 cm (median, 6 cm) Carney's triad (n = 1) Multifocal (n = 1) Recurrence or metastases involving liver (n = 9)	None (n = 13)	N/A	NED (n = 21) 7–41 y AWD (n = 5) 9–22 y DOD (n = 6) 95% presented with anemia and gastrointestinal bleeding.
Janeway[20,b]	27 6–22 (mean, 14) 23/4	N/A	N/A	Carney's triad (n = 2)	None (n = 24) KIT V559-560 exon 11 (n = 1) KIT AY 502-503 exon 9 (n = 1) PDGFR D842V exon 18 (n = 1)	N/A	N/A
Agaram[19]	17 8–17 (median, 14.5) 12/5	Stomach (n = 15) Omentum (n = 1) Small bowel (n = 1)	Epithelioid (n = 8) Spindle/epithelioid (n = 6) Spindle (n = 3) 1–76/50 HPF (median, 7)	Multifocal (n = 13) Carney's triad (n = 2) Peritoneal metastases (n = 9) Liver metastases (n = 5) Lymph node metastases (n = 4)	None (n = 15) KIT K557 exon 11 deletion (n = 1) PDGFR D842V exon 18 (n = 1)	Neoadjuvant imatinib (n = 6; 1 SD; 1 MR) Adjuvant imatinib (n = 1/NE) Sunitinib (n = 4; 1 SD; 1 MR) One patient received nilotinib with SD	NED (n = 6) 3–80 mo AWD (n = 8) 30–188 mo DOD (n = 1) 138 mo Mitotic activity did not correlate with clinical outcome. Mutations seen only in male patients.

Reference	n	Age (y) (median) M/F	Location	Histology/Mitosis	Size/Clinical	Mutation	Treatment	Outcome
Cypriano[10]	7	0.25–17 (median, 10.2) 4/3	Stomach (n = 2) Small intestine (n = 2) Colon (n = 2) Abdominal wall (n = 1)	Spindle (n = 5) Spindle/epithelioid (n = 1) Epithelioid (n = 1) 5–250 mitosis/HPF (median, 115/50 HPF)	Size <5 cm to 32 cm Local recurrence/progression (n = 3) Liver metastases (n = 1)	N/A	Adjuvant imatinib/NE	4 NED 1.3–12.7 y
Price[22]	6	6–14 (median, 13.6) 4/2	Stomach (n = 6)	Spindle/epithelioid (number not specified)	Carney's triad (n = 2) Multifocal (n = 3) Local recurrence (n = 1)	N/A (n = 3) No mutations (n = 2) KIT codon 456 exon 9 (n = 1)	N/A	NED (n = 4) Lost to F/U (n = 1) All patients presented with iron deficiency anemia and two had positive occult blood in stool. Endoscopic biopsies did not yield a diagnosis in these patients.
Kerr[44]	4	10–16 (median, 12) 4/0	Stomach (n = 4)	Spindle/epithelioid (n = 4) 2–28 mitosis /HPF	Size 3.8–8 cm (median, 6.5 cm) Multifocal (n = 4) Lymph nodes (n = 2) Local recurrence (n = 1)	N/A	N/A	4 NED 8–9 y Three patients presented with anemia and gastrointestinal symptoms and one with a palpable abdominal mass.

(continued on next page)

Table 2
(continued)

Study	Number of Patients, Age (y), Sex (F/M)	Location	Pathologic Subtype/Mitosis	Other Relevant Information	KIT/PDFGR Mutations	Imatinib or Sunitinib/ Evaluable Response	Outcome/Comments
Sauseng[47]	4 11, 13, 14, 16 3/1	Stomach (n = 4)	Epithelioid (n = 1) N/A (n = 3)	Carney-Stratakis (n = 1) Size 3.5–8 cm	N/A	Neoadjuvant imatinib (n = 1; 1 SD) Adjuvant imatinib (n = 1/NE)	NED 23 mo–10 y All patients presented with anemia, fatigue, and/or gastrointestinal bleeding.
Pasini[16]	2 9,13 0/2	Stomach (n = 1) N/A (n = 1)	N/A	One patient with multifocal disease Carney-Stratakis (n = 2) One patient a monozygotic twin	N/A	N/A	N/A
Muniyappa[48]	1 16 1/0	Stomach	Epithelioid	Size >6 cm Multifocal Liver metastases	N/A	Imatinib/PD	AWD 10 mo
Delemarre[25]	1 14 0/1	Stomach		Size 6 cm Liver and nodal metastases Carney's triad	No KIT or PDGFR mutations	Imatinib/1 PR	N/A

O'Sullivan[49]	1 11 1/0	Stomach	Spindle/ epithelioid <5/50 HPF	Size 3 cm Multifocal	No KIT or PDGFR mutations	N/A	NED 18 mo Patient presented with anemia and abdominal pain. Diagnosis was established by endoscopy.
Kuroiwa[21]	1 12 1/0	Stomach	N/A 8/50 HPF	Size 35 cm Multifocal	PDFGR codon 842 exon 18	Adjuvant imatinib/NE	NED 25 mo
Hayashi[50]	1 13 0/1	Stomach	Spindle/ epithelioid >5/10 HPF	Size 6 cm Liver metastases	N/A	Adjuvant imatinib/NE	NED 8 mo Patient presented with gastric bleeding and anemia.
Egloff[51]	1 8 1/0	Stomach	N/A	N/A	N/A	N/A	N/A Patient presented with gastrointestinal bleeding.
Iwasaki[52]	1 16 1/0	Stomach	Spindle <5/50 HPF	Size 7.5 cm	N/A	N/A	Unknown Patient presented with dizziness and anemia.
Chiarugi[23]	1 14 0/1	Duodenum	Spindle/ epithelioid <5/50 HPF	Size 4 cm	No KIT or PDGFR mutations	N/A	NED 24 mo Patient presented with anemia and upper gastrointestinal bleeding.

(continued on next page)

Table 2
(continued)

Study	Number of Patients, Age (y), Sex (F/M)	Location	Pathologic Subtype/Mitosis	Other Relevant Information	KIT/PDFGR Mutations	Imatinib or Sunitinib/ Evaluable Response	Outcome/Comments
Park[53]	1 / 11 / 0/1	Stomach	N/A	Size 10 cm Multifocal	N/A	N/A	NED 9 mo Patient presented with abdominal pain and anemia.
Raffensperger[54]	1 / 14 / 1/0	Stomach	Epithelioid 1–2 mitosis/HPF	Size 4.5 cm Multifocal Liver metastases Lymph node metastases Carney's triad	N/A	Adjuvant imatinib/NE	DOD 16 y Patient presented with anemia, pallor, and fatigue.
Terada[55]	1 / 4 / 1/0	Colon	Spindle/epitheliod 2 mitosis/10 HPF	Size 4.5 cm	N/A	N/A	NED 12 mo Patient presented with abdominal pain and constipation.
Wu[56]	1 / 0 / 0/1	Jejunum	Spindle <5/50 HPF	Size 3.5 cm	N/A	N/A	NED 12 mo Patient presented with abdominal distension and obstruction.
Mendes[57]	1 / 17 / 1/0	Stomach	Spindle/epithelioid 4/10 HPF	N/A Carney's triad	N/A	N/A	NED 5 y
Bates[58]	1 / 14 d / 1/0	Jejunum	1.5 cm Spindle and epithelioid 10/50 HPF	N/A	N/A	N/A	NED 12 mo Patient presented with intestinal obstruction.

Reference	No.	Age (mo)	M/F	Location	Histology	Size/Metastases	KIT mutation		Outcome/Comments
Li[32]	1	12	1/0	Stomach	8 cm, 5–6/50 HPF, Epithelioid	8 cm, Multinodular, Liver metastases	No KIT mutations	N/A	Unknown. Patient presented with anemia and diagnosis established by endoscopy.
Viola[59]	1	14	1/0	Small bowel	Spindle	Size 2.5 cm	N/A	N/A	NED 48 mo. Patient presented with anemia and occult blood in stool. Diagnosis made by wireless capsule endoscopy.
Gallegos-Castorena[60]	1	12	0/1	Ileum	5 cm, Spindle	Size 5 cm	N/A	N/A	NED 12 mo. Patient had previous history of osteosarcoma and presented with abdominal pain and weight loss.
Shenoy[61]	1	newborn	0/1	Ileum	Spindle, 1/10 HPF	2.5 cm	N/A	N/A	NED 12 mo. Patient presented with abdominal distension and delayed passage of meconium.

(continued on next page)

Table 2
(continued)

Study	Number of Patients, Age (y), Sex (F/M)	Location	Pathologic Subtype/Mitosis	Other Relevant Information	KIT/PDFGR Mutations	Imatinib or Sunitinib/ Evaluable Response	Outcome/Comments
Johnston[62]	1 17 1/0	Stomach	N/A	N/A	N/A	N/A	NED 13 mo Patient presented with anemia and a palpable abdominal mass, were unresponsive to preoperative chemotherapy with DTIC/doxorubicin, and had a previous history of neuroblastoma at 5 mo of age.
Murray[24]	1 15 1/0	Stomach	Spindle 1–2/10 HPF	N/A	No *KIT* or *PDGFR* mutations	Imatinib and sunitinib/SD	Unknown Patient presented with pallor, lethargy, and anemia.

Abbreviations: AWD, alive with disease; DOD, died of disease; F/U, follow-up; HPF, high power field; MR, mixed response; N/A, not available or not done; NE, not evaluable; NED, no evidence of disease; SD, stable disease.

a Included patients with gastric primaries only.

b This series included patients up to 24 years of age.

period. Two patients had a prior history of malignancy that included osteosarcoma and neuroblastoma. Twelve patients (10%) had a diagnosis of the Carney triad or Carney-Stratakis syndrome, emphasizing the need to search for features suggestive of these syndromes when initially evaluating pediatric patients with GIST. The GIST component of these syndromes usually presents with symptoms of anemia and gastrointestinal bleeding, whereas paragangliomas may elicit symptoms related to excess production of cathecolamines.[13,15]

Most patients with pediatric GIST present during the second decade of life; the median age at presentation in three large series was between 13 and 14.5 years.[11,19,20] Unlike adult sporadic GIST, pediatric GIST commonly affected females (89/121;74%), was associated with a higher proportion of tumors located in the stomach (79/93;85%), had a predominance of epithelioid (34/78;44%) or epithelioid/spindle cell morphology (22/78;28%), and rarely had *KIT* or *PDGFR* mutations. The reported tumor size varied widely (**Fig. 1**) and reached dimensions of up to 35 cm in one patient.[21] The mitotic rate ranged from 0 to 250; however, there was a lack of uniformity when reporting the number of high-power fields, which ranged from 10 to 50. In two series, the mitotic rate and the size of the tumor were not predictive of clinical behavior when adult reporting criteria were applied. These findings suggest that pediatric GIST has a somewhat unpredictable clinical course, and that patients may be more prone to have metastases regardless of the prognostic criteria used in adults, such as tumor site, size, and mitotic rate.[6,9,19,22] Another distinct feature of pediatric GIST is the presence of multifocality, which was reported in 28 of the patients (23%) depicted in **Table 2** and in 13 of 16 patients in one large series.[19] The presence of multiple tumor foci within an anatomic region may account for the high incidence of local recurrences as a result of incomplete tumor resection in these patients. The dramatic resemblance in clinical presentation, such as female predominance, multifocality, an indolent clinical course, and a lack of *KIT* or *PDGFR* mutations, between pediatric GIST and other syndromes such as NF-1, the Carney triad, and Carney-Stratakis dyad suggests that there might be a possible pathogenic link and requires further study.

PROGNOSIS

Pediatric GIST has an indolent clinical course. Despite the fact that many patients develop multiple disease recurrences spanning over many years or present with

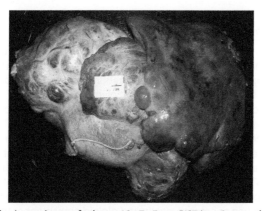

Fig. 1. Gross pathologic specimen of a large 10×7×5 cm GIST in a 9-year-old child. No *PDGFR* or *KIT* mutations were present in the resected gastric tumor. Despite the size, a complete resection was possible without compromising gastric function.

metastatic disease most commonly affecting the local tumor bed, lymph nodes, peritoneum, and liver, few have died of their disease. In one of the largest series of pediatric GIST reported to date, 10 of 12 patients (83%) had metastatic disease yet only one died as a consequence of this tumor.[19] Another large series with longer follow-up supports the assertion that pediatric GIST has an indolent course but also suggests that some patients will eventually succumb to the disease.[11] In this series, six patients died of disease after surviving a median of 16 years from the time of diagnosis.[11] These observations have important clinical implications for primary therapy, because extensive or disabling surgeries might not be indicated as a primary form of treatment for these patients (see management guidelines).

BIOLOGY OF PEDIATRIC GASTROINTESTINAL STROMAL TUMORS

Basic research on the biology of pediatric GIST has been hampered by the rarity of the disease and the lack of preclinical models. Despite these limitations, knowledge gained from the study of adult GIST and related tumor types (eg, paragangliomas) and the advent of newer research techniques (eg, expression and single nucleotide polymorphism arrays) have allowed for significant progress in the understanding of this rare and challenging pediatric entity.

Receptor Tyrosine Kinase Mutations

As mentioned previously, KIT and PDGFRA mutations are rare in pediatric patients with GIST. Among the 64 pediatric GISTs subjected to mutational testing and reported in the literature (**Table 2**), only 7 (11%) had a KIT or PDGFRA mutation.[11,19-25] Interestingly, these mutations were evenly distributed in exons 11 and 9 of the KIT proto-oncogene, and PDFGR mutations were relatively common, seen in three of the seven reported cases. This pattern is different from that seen in adults with sporadic GIST, in which KIT mutations are 10 times more common than PDGFRA mutations.[1] In pediatric GIST, these mutations are more often encountered in males. In fact, only one female patient aged less than 18 years with a PDGFRA mutation has been reported.[21] Although one could hypothesize that there are KIT and PDGFRA mutations in pediatric GIST that are located in different exons than those described in adults and are thus not sequenced in routine mutation analysis, no novel KIT mutations were identified when full coding length KIT sequencing from cDNA was performed in 11 pediatric GIST tumors.[19,20]

Genetic Mechanisms of Progression

Following receptor tyrosine kinase mutation, adult GIST undergoes a typical progression of chromosomal changes that can be detected by traditional cytogenetic analysis,[26,27] comparative genomic hybridization (CGH),[28-30] fluorescence in situ hybridization (FISH),[31] or single nucleotide polymorphism (SNP)[20] analysis. Similar chromosomal regions are affected in most adult GISTs regardless of whether the initiating receptor tyrosine kinase mutation is in KIT or PDGFRA.[26,29] The typically affected regions include 1p, 14q, 22q, and 9p,[26-31] and these chromosomal changes contribute to clinical progression. Loss of 14q and 22q loss is present in low- and high-grade GIST, whereas 1p and 9p loss occurs in more advanced GIST. Surprisingly, most pediatric GISTs lacking KIT or PDGFRA mutations (wild-type GIST) have minimal large scale chromosomal changes. By 10K SNP analysis, 12 of 13 pediatric wild-type GISTs had preservation of heterozygosity and diploid copy number throughout the entire genome.[20] Prior evaluations of GIST in pediatric patients using conventional cytogenetics have shown normal (diploid) karyotypes.[14,32] By CGH analysis, 60% of 13 wild-type GISTs occurring in pediatric patients with the Carney triad lacked chromosomal changes. Among the 40% of tumors with chromosomal changes, the most commonly identified abnormality was 1q deletion, seen in three GISTs; 1q contains the gene for SDHC discussed later.[14]

Gene Expression

In gene expression microarray experiments, pediatric wild-type GIST clusters distinctly from adult wild-type GIST and adult gastric GIST (95% of which have *KIT* or *PDGFRA* mutations).[19] GISTs occurring in young adults that have features similar to those seen in pediatric patients (multifocality, epithelioid morphology, and indolent course) have gene expression profiles that more closely resemble pediatric wild-type GIST.[19] Genes distinguishing pediatric wild-type GIST from adult wild-type GIST and adult gastric GIST include those for cytokine receptor-like factor 1 (CRLF1), fibroblast growth factor 4 (FGF4), brain and acute leukemia cytoplasmic (BAALC), pleomorphic adenoma gene 1 (PLAG1), and insulin-like growth factor 1 receptor (IGF1R).[19] The gene expression array experiments described previously were performed using a small number of tumor samples, and the results have not been confirmed by other groups due to the difficulty in obtaining fresh frozen samples suitable for RNA extraction in such a rare tumor.

KIT as a Potential Therapeutic Target

Although *KIT* generally lacks transforming mutations in pediatric GIST, it is expressed and activated in pediatric wild-type GIST.[19,20,33] Surprisingly, the extent of *KIT* activation in pediatric wild-type GIST is similar to that seen in adult *KIT*-mutant GIST.[19,20] The signaling intermediates downstream of *KIT*, mitogen activated protein kinase (MAPK), Akt, S6, and mTOR, are also activated in pediatric GIST.[19,20] These data suggest that *KIT* and downstream signaling intermediates may be reasonable therapeutic targets for pediatric patients with GIST. Small molecule inhibitors of *KIT* include imatinib (Gleevec), sorafenib (Nexavar), sunitinib (Sutent), nilotinib (Tasigna), and dasatinib (Sprycel). The potency of these molecules to inhibit wild-type *KIT* is not equivalent. When assayed in vitro in Ba/F3 cells stably expressing wild-type *KIT*, imatinib is the least potent with an IC_{50} of 3132 nmol/L, and nilotinib, dasatinib, and sorafinib are the most potent with an IC_{50} of 27, 44, and 66 nmol/L, respectively.[19]

Insulin-Like Growth Factor 1 Receptor

Expression of IGF1R is five times higher in pediatric wild-type GIST than in adult wild-type GIST.[19] The insulin-like growth factor 1 (IGF1) and its receptor, IGF1R, are central mediators of cellular growth and proliferation and normal growth and development as evidenced by the fact that mice lacking the IGF1R are half the size of normal mice.[34] An analysis of IGF1R protein expression in GIST by western blotting and immunohistochemistry shows that IGF1R is expressed in all GIST[35] but that levels of expression are much higher in wild-type GIST.[36] In the only published study of pediatric wild-type GIST in which IGF1R protein expression was evaluated, IGF1R expression was elevated to a similar degree as seen in adult wild-type GIST.[36] IGF1R is activated in most GISTs, but levels of activation do not correlate with the amount of total IGF1R expression.[36] High IGF1R expression in wild-type GIST is partially due to IGF1R gene amplification, which was present in 70% of wild-type GISTs and 30% of *KIT/PDGFRA*-mutant GISTs examined.[37] Importantly, during IGF1 stimulation, inhibition of IGF1R by a small molecule inhibitor decreased proliferation of a *KIT*-mutant GIST cell line, and co-administration of imatinib had an additive effect.[36] Braconi and colleagues[35] have also reported that IGF1 and IGF2 are variably expressed in GIST and that higher levels of tumor IGF1 expression correlate with a poorer clinical outcome. These findings strongly argue in favor of pursuing the IGF1R as a therapeutic target in pediatric GIST.

Succinate Dehydrogenase and the Carney-Stratakis Syndrome

Germline mutations in the *SDHB*, *SDHC*, and *SDHD* genes are known to result in hereditary paragangliomas and pheochromocytomas,[37–39] and germline mutations or deletions in *SDHB*, *SDHC*, or *SDHD* are present in the majority of patients with the Carney-Stratakis syndrome.[16,17,40] Mutations or deletions involving *SDHB* are the most common, found in 4 of 9 families and 5 of 11 patients, followed by *SDHC* mutations present in 2 of 9 families and 2 of 11 patients, and *SDHD* mutations found in 1 of 9 families and 1 of 11 patients.[16]

Several recent reviews provide an in depth discussion of the mechanisms by which mutations in the genes for SDH lead to cancer susceptibility.[41,42] In hereditary pheochromocytoma and paraganglioma, SDH acts as a typical tumor suppressor gene.[41] In three GISTs from patients with Carney-Stratakis syndrome caused by germline SDH mutations, loss of the functional allele was documented, suggesting that SDH may act as a tumor suppressor gene in Carney-Stratakis syndrome associated with GIST as well.[16]

Whether SDH mutations are present in pediatric wild-type GISTs occurring in patients without an apparent family or personal history suggestive of Carney-Stratakis syndrome is an area of active research. An additional area of great interest is the extent to which SDH dysfunction is present in *KIT/PDGFRA*-mutant GISTs, GISTs arising in Carney triad patients, and adult wild-type GISTs. As mentioned previously, a subset of GISTs from patients with the Carney triad have deletion of the region containing *SDHC*.[14] *SDHB* maps to 1p36, and loss of 1p is relatively common in more advanced *KIT/PDGFRA*-mutant GISTs.[27,29–31] In a recent abstract, loss of heterozygosity at the *SDHB* loci was detected in 50% of GIST cases and loss of heterozygosity at the *SDHC* and *SDHD* loci were detected at a lower frequency.[43] Whether the genomic losses at *SDHB*, *SDHC*, and *SDHD* seen in *KIT/PDGFRA*-mutant GIST, adult wild-type GISTs, and GISTs arising in Carney triad patients are related to oncogenesis is not yet known.

EVALUATION AND WORK-UP

There are no published guidelines for the management of pediatric GIST, and the management guidelines herein are offered recognizing that, given the available published literature, recommendations are based on nonanalytic case series and expert opinion. **Fig. 2** summarizes the authors' suggested recommendations for the evaluation and diagnosis of these patients. Given its rarity and complexity, all children with suspected GIST should be managed by a team with expertise in sarcoma. Particular attention should be paid to the family history, prior history of malignancy, and symptoms of bleeding, anemia, abdominal pain, abdominal distension, hyperpigmentation, and catecholamine excess. Laboratory evaluations should include a complete blood count, reticulocyte count, and serum and liver chemistries. Initial anatomic evaluation of the tumor should include a chest radiograph (searching for pulmonary chondromas), a CT of the abdomen and pelvis, and, in selected cases, an endoscopy. Referral to an experienced surgeon preferably with expertise in the management of patients with sarcoma or GIST is recommended. Depending on the family history, they also may need to be assessed by an experienced geneticist.

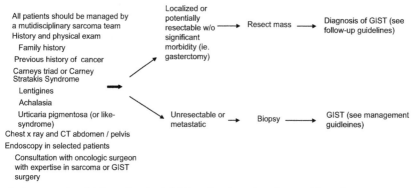

Fig. 2. Suggested guidelines for the initial evaluation of patients with pediatric GIST.

MANAGEMENT AND FOLLOW-UP

Once the diagnosis of GIST has been established, all samples should be subjected to mutational analysis (**Figs. 3** and **4**). If *KIT* or *PDGFR* mutations are detected, one should follow the guidelines published by the National Comprehensive Cancer Network for adult GIST (http://www.nccn.org/professionals/physician_gls/PDF/sarcoma.pdf). If no mutations are detected and the tumor is localized and resectable without significant morbidity (ie, total gastrectomy), surgical resection of the mass is recommended with the goal of achieving negative surgical margins. Although lymph node sampling is not recommended for patients with adult GIST, pediatric GIST is associated with a relatively high incidence of lymph node metastases;[19,44] therefore, any abnormal lymphatic chains identified at the time of surgery should be resected and submitted for pathologic examination. If all tumor has been resected, follow-up should include physical examination, a complete blood count, chest radiography, and CT of the abdomen and pelvis at

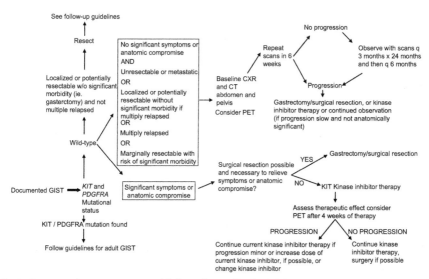

Fig. 3. Suggested management guidelines for pediatric GIST.

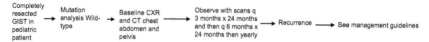

Fig. 4. Suggested follow-up guidelines for pediatric GIST.

3-month intervals for 24 months, followed by visits at 6-month intervals for 24 months and yearly thereafter.

For patients with unresectable or metastatic disease who are clinically asymptomatic, the authors recommend a set of baseline images including a chest radiograph and CT of the abdomen and pelvis and possibly positron emission tomography followed by repeat imaging in 6 weeks to assess the rate of tumor growth. If the patient is clinically stable and the tumor has remained stable in size, future imaging should follow the same intervals described previously. If significant progression develops at any time or the patient becomes clinically symptomatic, surgical resection of the primary tumor is recommended; if this is not feasible, institution of kinase inhibitor therapy should be promptly initiated. A similar management approach is recommended for patients with indolent multiply recurrent tumors who are asymptomatic and for those in which the initial results of surgical resection are expected to yield an incomplete resection or an inadequate functional outcome.

For patients who experience clinical symptoms or significant progression, the authors recommend surgical resection of the tumor even if it entails a total gastrectomy. If after consultation with an experienced surgeon it is apparent that surgical resection is not feasible, kinase inhibitor therapy should be initiated. It is not clear what the optimal front-line medical therapy should be for these patients. A review of 16 children and adolescents treated with various tyrosine kinase inhibitors is summarized in **Table 2**. Imatinib was administered in the neoadjuvant setting to 10 patients, with one partial response and three stable diseases observed. Sunitinib was administered to five patients with no significant objective responses; however, in a separate report not included in **Table 2**, Janeway and collaborators[45] described one patient with a partial response and five with disease stabilization that lasted from 7 to 18 months following the administration of sunitinib in seven patients who failed imatinib. Nilotinib was used in only one of patients, and the best response observed was stable disease.[19]

Based on these observations, the authors recommend imatinib as the first drug of choice to be used in the neoadjuvant setting at a dose of 230 mg/m^2 up to a maximum of 400 mg per day.[46] If future response assessment shows disease stabilization, this therapy and dose should be continued. If progression develops, an increase in the dose of imatinib to 600 or 800 mg per day (in adult-sized patients), a switch to another kinase inhibitor such as sunitinib or nilotinib, or enrollment in a clinical trial that incorporates novel treatments such as IGF1R inhibitors should be considered.

FUTURE RESEARCH

Much remains to be learned about the natural history, optimal management, and biology of pediatric GIST. The development of a registration trial with well-annotated samples is urgently needed to enhance our ability to study the biology of and develop more effective therapies for pediatric GIST. In an important step toward a national registration trial, the National Institutes of Health has recently developed an initiative to study pediatric GIST which includes a pediatric GIST clinic. This multidisciplinary clinic which convenes twice yearly brings together pediatric and adult oncologists, surgeons, and geneticists who carefully review and capture clinical and laboratory information from significant numbers of pediatric patients with GIST. It is expected that this initiative will lead to a better understanding of the clinical and laboratory features of pediatric GIST. Priorities for biologic studies of pediatric GIST include the creation of a preclinical in vitro or in vivo model of the disease, further examination of the role of the IGF system in pediatric GIST oncogenesis, and evaluation of whether SDH mutations or other genetic alterations in SDH are present in pediatric GIST. Based on the laboratory observations described earlier, a phase II study of IGF1R monoclonal antibody therapy for pediatric wild-type GIST is being developed in collaboration with the Sarcoma Alliance for Research through Collaboration.

SUMMARY

Pediatric GISTs are different from adult GISTs and are characterized by female predominance, epithelioid histology, gastric location, a paucity of *KIT* or *PDGFRA* mutations, an indolent clinical course, and minimal response to tyrosine kinase inhibitors. Efforts to better study this disease are being undertaken and will likely lead to new treatment approaches for these patients.

REFERENCES

1. Corless CL, Fletcher JA, Heinrich MC. Biology of gastrointestinal stromal tumors. J Clin Oncol 2004;22:3813–25.
2. Tryggvason G, Gislason HG, Magnusson MK, et al. Gastrointestinal stromal tumors in Iceland, 1990–2003: the Icelandic GIST study, a population-based incidence and pathologic risk stratification study. Int J Cancer 2005;117:289–93.
3. Nilsson B, Bumming P, Meis-Kindblom JM, et al. Gastrointestinal stromal tumors: the incidence, prevalence, clinical course, and prognostication in the preimatinib mesylate era–a population-based study in western Sweden. Cancer 2005;103: 821–9.
4. Perez EA, Livingstone AS, Franceschi D, et al. Current incidence and outcomes of gastrointestinal mesenchymal tumors including gastrointestinal stromal tumors. J Am Coll Surg 2006;202:623–9.
5. Rubin BP. Gastrointestinal stromal tumours: an update. Histopathology 2006;48: 83–96.
6. Miettinen M, Lasota J. Gastrointestinal stromal tumors: review of morphology, molecular pathology, prognosis and differential diagnosis. Arch Pathol Lab Med 2006;130:1466–78.
7. Demetri GD, van Oosterom AT, Garrett CR, et al. Efficacy and safety of sunitinib in patients with advanced gastrointestinal stromal tumour after failure of imatinib: a randomised controlled trial. Lancet 2006;368:1329–38.
8. Demetri GD, von Mehren M, Blanke CD, et al. Efficacy and safety of imatinib mesylate in advanced gastrointestinal stromal tumors. N Engl J Med 2002;347: 472–80.
9. Fletcher CD, Berman JJ, Corless C, et al. Diagnosis of gastrointestinal stromal tumors: a consensus approach. Hum Pathol 2002;33:459–65.
10. Cypriano MS, Jenkins JJ, Pappo AS, et al. Pediatric gastrointestinal stromal tumors and leiomyosarcoma. Cancer 2004;101:39–50.
11. Miettinen M, Lasota J, Sobin LH. Gastrointestinal stromal tumors of the stomach in children and young adults: a clinicopathologic, immunohistochemical, and molecular genetic study of 44 cases with long-term follow-up and review of the literature. Am J Surg Pathol 2005;29:1373–81.

12. Prakash S, Sarran L, Socci N, et al. Gastrointestinal stromal tumors in children and young adults: a clinicopathologic, molecular, and genomic study of 15 cases and review of the literature. J Pediatr Hematol Oncol 2005;27:179–87.

13. Carney JA. Gastric stromal sarcoma, pulmonary chondroma, and extra-adrenal paraganglioma (Carney triad): natural history, adrenocortical component, and possible familial occurrence. Mayo Clin Proc 1999;74:543–52.

14. Matyakhina L, Bei TA, McWhinney SR, et al. Genetics of Carney triad: recurrent losses at chromosome 1 but lack of germline mutations in genes associated with paragangliomas and gastrointestinal stromal tumors. J Clin Endocrinol Metab 2007;92:2938–43.

15. Carney JA, Stratakis CA. Familial paraganglioma and gastric stromal sarcoma: a new syndrome distinct from the Carney triad. Am J Med Genet 2002;108:132–9.

16. Pasini B, McWhinney SR, Bei T, et al. Clinical and molecular genetics of patients with the Carney-Stratakis syndrome and germline mutations of the genes coding for the succinate dehydrogenase subunits SDHB, SDHC, and SDHD. Eur J Hum Genet 2008;16:79–88.

17. McWhinney SR, Pasini B, Stratakis CA. Familial gastrointestinal stromal tumors and germ-line mutations. N Engl J Med 2007;357:1054–6.

18. Li FP, Fletcher JA, Heinrich MC, et al. Familial gastrointestinal stromal tumor syndrome: phenotypic and molecular features in a kindred. J Clin Oncol 2005;23:2735–43.

19. Agaram NP, Laquaglia MP, Ustun B, et al. Molecular characterization of pediatric gastrointestinal stromal tumors. Clin Cancer Res 2008;14:3204–15.

20. Janeway KA, Liegl B, Harlow A, et al. Pediatric KIT wild-type and platelet-derived growth factor receptor alpha wild-type gastrointestinal stromal tumors share KIT activation but not mechanisms of genetic progression with adult gastrointestinal stromal tumors. Cancer Res 2007;67:9084–8.

21. Kuroiwa M, Hiwatari M, Hirato J, et al. Advanced-stage gastrointestinal stromal tumor treated with imatinib in a 12-year-old girl with a unique mutation of PDGFRA. J Pediatr Surg 2005;40:1798–801.

22. Price VE, Zielenska M, Chilton-MacNeill S, et al. Clinical and molecular characteristics of pediatric gastrointestinal stromal tumors (GISTs). Pediatr Blood Cancer 2005;45:20–4.

23. Chiarugi M, Galatioto C, Lippolis P, et al. Gastrointestinal stromal tumour of the duodenum in childhood: a rare case report. BMC Cancer 2007;7:79.

24. Murray M, Hatcher H, Jessop F, et al. Treatment of wild-type gastrointestinal stromal tumor (WT-GIST) with imatinib and sunitinib. Pediatr Blood Cancer 2008;50:386–8.

25. Delemarre L, Aronson D, van Rijn R, et al. Respiratory symptoms in a boy revealing Carney triad. Pediatr Blood Cancer 2008;50:399–401.

26. Heinrich MC, Corless CL, Duensing A, et al. PDGFRA activating mutations in gastrointestinal stromal tumors. Science 2003;299:708–10.

27. Heinrich MC, Rubin BP, Longley BJ, et al. Biology and genetic aspects of gastrointestinal stromal tumors: KIT activation and cytogenetic alterations. Hum Pathol 2002;33:484–95.

28. Kim NG, Kim JJ, Ahn JY, et al. Putative chromosomal deletions on 9P, 9Q and 22Q occur preferentially in malignant gastrointestinal stromal tumors. Int J Cancer 2000;85:633–8.

29. Wozniak A, Sciot R, Guillou L, et al. Array CGH analysis in primary gastrointestinal stromal tumors: cytogenetic profile correlates with anatomic site and tumor aggressiveness, irrespective of mutational status. Genes Chromosomes Cancer 2007;46:261–76.

30. El-Rifai W, Sarlomo-Rikala M, Andersson LC, et al. DNA sequence copy number changes in gastrointestinal stromal tumors: tumor progression and prognostic significance. Cancer Res 2000;60:3899–903.
31. Debiec-Rychter M, Lasota J, Sarlomo-Rikala M, et al. Chromosomal aberrations in malignant gastrointestinal stromal tumors: correlation with c-KIT gene mutation. Cancer Genet Cytogenet 2001;128:24–30.
32. Li P, Wei J, West AB, et al. Epithelioid gastrointestinal stromal tumor of the stomach with liver metastases in a 12-year-old girl: aspiration cytology and molecular study. Pediatr Dev Pathol 2002;5:386–94.
33. Agaram NP, Besmer P, Wong GC, et al. Pathologic and molecular heterogeneity in imatinib-stable or imatinib-responsive gastrointestinal stromal tumors. Clin Cancer Res 2007;13:170–81.
34. Liu JP, Baker J, Perkins AS, et al. Mice carrying null mutations of the genes encoding insulin-like growth factor I (IGF-1) and type 1 IGF receptor (IGF1R). Cell 1993;75:59–72.
35. Braconi C, Bracci R, Bearzi I, et al. Insulin-like growth factor (IGF) 1 and 2 help to predict disease outcome in GIST patients. Ann Oncol 2008;19:1293–8.
36. Tarn C, Rink L, Merkel E, et al. Insulin-like growth factor 1 receptor is a potential therapeutic target for gastrointestinal stromal tumors. Proc Natl Acad Sci USA 2008;105:8387–92.
37. Baysal BE, Ferrell RE, Willett-Brozick JE, et al. Mutations in SDHD, a mitochondrial complex II gene, in hereditary paraganglioma. Science 2000;287:848–51.
38. Niemann S, Muller U. Mutations in SDHC cause autosomal dominant paraganglioma, type 3. Nat Genet 2000;26:268–70.
39. Astuti D, Douglas F, Lennard TW, et al. Germline SDHD mutation in familial phaeochromocytoma. Lancet 2001;357:1181–2.
40. Bolland M, Benn D, Croxson M, et al. Gastrointestinal stromal tumour in succinate dehydrogenase subunit B mutation-associated familial phaeochromocytoma/paraganglioma. ANZ J Surg 2006;76:763–4.
41. Gottlieb E, Tomlinson IP. Mitochondrial tumour suppressors: a genetic and biochemical update. Nat Rev Cancer 2005;5:857–66.
42. King A, Selak MA, Gottlieb E. Succinate dehydrogenase and fumarate hydratase: linking mitochondrial dysfunction and cancer. Oncogene 2006;25:4675–82.
43. Ferrando B, Pappi P, Bonello L, et al. Somatic loss of heterozygosity or allelic imbalance at succinate dehydrogenase B, C and D loci in sporadic GISTs. In: Proceedings of the American Association for Cancer Research Annual Meeting, Los Angeles, California, April 2007.
44. Kerr JZ, Hicks MJ, Nuchtern JG, et al. Gastrointestinal autonomic nerve tumors in the pediatric population: a report of four cases and a review of the literature. Cancer 1999;85:220–30.
45. Janeway KA, Albritton KH, Van den Abele AD, et al. Sunitinib treatment in pediatric patients with advanced GIST following failure of imatinib. Pediatr Blood Ca; in press.
46. Champagne MA, Capdeville R, Krailo M, et al. Imatinib mesylate (STI571) for treatment of children with Philadelphia chromosome-positive leukemia: results from a Children's Oncology Group phase 1 study. Blood 2004;104:2655–60.
47. Sauseng W, Benesch M, Lackner H, et al. Clinical, radiological, and pathological findings in four children with gastrointestinal stromal tumors of the stomach. Pediatr Hematol Oncol 2007;24:209–19.
48. Muniyappa P, Kay M, Feinberg L, et al. The endoscopic appearance of a gastrointestinal stromal tumor in a pediatric patient. J Pediatr Surg 2007;42:1302–5.

49. O'Sullivan MJ, McCabe A, Gillett P, et al. Multiple gastric stromal tumors in a child without syndromic association lacks common KIT or PDGFR alpha mutations. Pediatr Dev Pathol 2005;8:685–9.
50. Hayashi Y, Okazaki T, Yamataka A, et al. Gastrointestinal stromal tumor in a child and review of the literature. Pediatr Surg Int 2005;21:914–7.
51. Egloff A, Lee EY, Dillon JE. Gastrointestinal stromal tumor (GIST) of stomach in a pediatric patient. Pediatr Radiol 2005;35:728–9.
52. Iwasaki M, Morimoto T, Sano K, et al. A case of pediatric gastrointestinal stromal tumor of the stomach. Pediatr Int 2005;47:102–4.
53. Park J, Rubinas TC, Fordham LA, et al. Multifocal gastrointestinal stromal tumor (GIST) of the stomach in an 11-year-old girl. Pediatr Radiol 2006;36:1212–4.
54. Raffensperger J, Krueger R. Carney's triad: a 16-year follow-up. J Pediatr Surg 2007;42:1452–3.
55. Terada R, Ito S, Akama F, et al. Clinical and histopathological features of colonic stromal tumor in a child. J Gastroenterol 2000;35:456–9.
56. Wu SS, Buchmiller TL, Close P, et al. Congenital gastrointestinal pacemaker cell tumor. Arch Pathol Lab Med 1999;123:842–5.
57. Mendes W, Ayoub A, Chapchap P, et al. Association of gastrointestinal stromal tumor (leiomyosarcoma), pulmonary chondroma, and nonfunctional retroperitoneal paraganglioma. Med Pediatr Oncol 1998;31:537–40.
58. Bates AW, Feakins RM, Scheimberg I. Congenital gastrointestinal stromal tumour is morphologically indistinguishable from the adult form, but does not express CD117 and carries a favourable prognosis. Histopathology 2000;37:316–22.
59. Viola S, Dray X, Boudjemaa S, et al. Pediatric jejunal gastrointestinal stromal tumor diagnosed by wireless capsule endoscopy. J Pediatr Gastroenterol Nutr 2007;45:358–60.
60. Gallegos-Castorena S, Martinez-Avalos A, Francisco Ortiz de la OE, et al. Gastrointestinal stromal tumor in a patient surviving osteosarcoma. Med Pediatr Oncol 2003;40:338–9.
61. Shenoy MU, Singh SJ, Robson K, et al. Gastrointestinal stromal tumor: a rare cause of neonatal intestinal obstruction. Med Pediatr Oncol 2000;34:70–1.
62. Johnston DL, Olson JM, Benjamin DR. Gastrointestinal stromal tumor in a patient with previous neuroblastoma. J Pediatr Hematol Oncol 2001;23:255–6.

Imaging of Gastrointestinal Stromal Tumors and Assessment of Benefit from Systemic Therapy

Piyaporn Boonsirikamchai, MD, Donald A. Podoloff, MD,
Haesun Choi, MD*

KEYWORDS

- Gastrointestinal stromal tumors • Imaging
- Computed tomography

Gastrointestinal stromal tumor (GIST) accounts for only 0.2% of all gastrointestinal (GI) neoplasm[1] but is the most common tumor of nonepithelial origin in the GI tract, with an overall incidence of 3,000 to 5,000 cases per year in the United States.[2–4] The term "gastrointestinal stromal tumor" was first used by Mazur and Clark[5] to describe an unusual type of nonepithelial GI tumor that lacked the traditional features of smooth muscle or Schwann cells. GISTs are now thought to derive from a precursor of the interstitial cells of Cajal, which are normally present in the myenteric plexus and are clearly distinct from other mesenchymal tumors, such as leiomyomas and leiomyosarcomas.[6] The interstitial cells of Cajal normally express a transmembrane receptor tyrosine kinase encoded by the *KIT* gene.[7] Almost all GISTs express activating mutations in *KIT* that lead to ligand-dependent *KIT* tyrosine kinase activation and promote tumor survival and growth.[8] Identifying *KIT* (CD117) is the key to making a diagnosis of GIST in 95% of patients. The small numbers of GIST patients whose tumors do not express detectable *KIT* mutations instead express activating mutations in the related tyrosine kinase platelet-derived growth factor receptor-alpha (*PDGFR-α*).[9]

For localized primary GISTs, surgical resection is the mainstay of therapy.[10] It is now well known that advanced GIST can be treated with a tyrosine kinase inhibitor imatinib (Gleevec; Novartis Pharma AG, Basel, Switzerland), with a remarkable response[11–13] and prolonged survival.[14,15] New second-line targeted agents are now also available for those with imatinib-resistant GISTs.[16] Definitive diagnosis thus is now particularly

Department of Diagnostic Radiology, The University of Texas M.D. Anderson Cancer Center, 1515 Holcombe Boulevard, Houston, TX 77030, USA
* Corresponding author.
E-mail address: hchoi@mdanderson.org (H. Choi).

Hematol Oncol Clin N Am 23 (2009) 35–48
doi:10.1016/j.hoc.2008.12.001
0889-8588/08/$ – see front matter © 2009 Elsevier Inc. All rights reserved.

important so that we can take advantage of these new highly effective molecularly targeted treatments. For KIT-negative GISTs, a tumor genotype assay to determine the mutational status of both the *KIT* and *PDGFR-α* genes is recommended to establish a definitive diagnosis.[17]

While GISTs have been increasingly recognized with the prolonged survival resulting from a combination of increasing numbers of diagnosis and highly effective new targeted treatments, the role of imaging has become more important not only for diagnosing and staging the tumors, but also for monitoring the effects of treatment and detecting tumor progression. Computed tomography (CT) is currently the modality of choice for these purposes, although other imaging techniques, such as fluorine-18-fluorodeoxyglucose (FDG) positron emission tomography (PET), MRI, and ultrasonography, can also be used. FDG-PET is highly sensitive in detecting GISTs and evaluating their response to treatment,[18,19] but access to PET imaging is still limited worldwide and technically challenging to reproduce between institutions. Additionally, in a small number of lesions, glucose uptake by GISTs before treatment is insufficient for detection by FDG-PET.[20] MRI is indicated for surgical planning in cases of localized rectal GISTs, for evaluation of liver lesions indeterminate on CT, and for cases in which CT is contraindicated. Ultrasonography, in expert hands, may also be useful to evaluate the liver.

This article reviews the role of different imaging modalities in the management of GISTs, with a focus on the assessment of benefit from systemic therapy.

COMPUTED TOMOGRAPHY

CT is widely accepted in general practice worldwide, and it is relatively simple to acquire the images. CT is reasonably reproducible, with no significant technical obstacles. CT is often the initial imaging modality used to evaluate patients presenting with nonspecific abdominal symptoms or a palpable abdominal mass. In patients with biopsy-proven GISTs, CT is the imaging modality of choice at initial presentation, for staging, and for monitoring the disease during its course.

Typically, CT images of the abdomen and pelvis are acquired before and following bolus administration (injection rate of no less than 3 cc per second) of an iodinated intravenous contrast agent and oral and rectal contrast agents. For contrast-enhanced CT, arterial- and portal-venous-phase images (obtained using a biphasic or triphasic technique) are required to optimize the detection and characterization of the hepatic metastasis or hypervascular masses, such as GISTs. The pattern and degree of enhancement are used to characterize the masses and to identify viable tumor tissues.

Perfusion CT may be used in patients with GIST in response evaluation[21] or detection of tumor recurrence after targeted therapy.[22] CT perfusion study is designed to evaluate tissue angiogenesis that can reflect the tumor viability and requires very fast data acquisition (eg, 0.5 seconds per image) following a fast bolus administration (injection rate of $\geq$ 5 cc per second) of intravenous contrast. This technique can provide quantitative data for angiogenic features, such as blood flow and volume, using a deconvolution-based method or a compartmental kinetic model.[23]

Initial Evaluation

GISTs are highly vascular submucosal masses and typically grow outward, away from the originating bowel lumen. At the time of presentation, the masses are often large or even massive, but bowel obstruction is rare. Despite their large size, the masses usually only displace adjacent organs and anatomic structures and direct invasion is rare, only being observed in advanced disease. Identifying the origin of the mass on CT images can often be challenging.

The CT features of GISTs can vary depending on the size, location, and aggressiveness of tumor. As in the case of other hypervascular masses, GISTs are visualized as enhancing solid masses and tumor vessels are often noted on enhanced CT images (**Fig. 1**). The primary GIST can occasionally present with ulceration and a fistula to the originating bowel lumen. Air or oral contrast agent may be seen within the fistularized mass on the CT images. In general, small tumors are found incidentally either by endoscopy or CT. If the tumor is incidentally found by endoscopy, CT should be performed to evaluate extraluminal extension. Small GISTs typically appear as well-defined soft-tissue, relatively low-density masses that appear relatively homogeneous on enhanced CT images. When the masses are large (usually >10 cm), they are often heterogeneous because of necrosis, hemorrhage, and myxoid degeneration. Calcification is rare.

Nearly 50% of patients with GISTs present with metastasis.[24] Metastasis in GISTs is hematogeneous. Unlike gastrointestinal adenocarcinomas, GISTs rarely metastasize to regional lymph nodes. The most common sites of metastases are the liver (**Fig. 2**) and peritoneum (**Fig. 3**). Less frequently, metastases can be found in the soft tissue, lung, and pleura. These metastatic lesions have CT features similar to those of the primary tumors: they may be (depending on the tumor size) homogeneously to heterogeneously enhancing soft-tissue masses, often with tumor vessels visible (see **Figs. 2** and **3**).

Response Evaluation

In patients who have undergone surgical resection of GISTs, CT is performed for surveillance of metastatic or recurrent disease after surgery. In patients with unresectable advanced disease or metastasis, CT is an excellent imaging modality for disease monitoring. The National Comprehensive Cancer Network recommends a follow-up CT scan every 3 to 6 months after surgical resection and within 3 months of the systemic treatment's initiation in patients with unresectable disease.[10]

Responding GISTs are characterized by a dramatic change in the pattern of enhancement on contrast-enhanced CT images, from heterogeneous hyper-attenuation to homogeneous hypo-attenuation, accompanying the resolution of enhancing tumor nodules and a decrease in tumor vessels, regardless of whether the tumor size decreases (see **Figs. 2** and **3**). These changes can be observed within 1 or 2

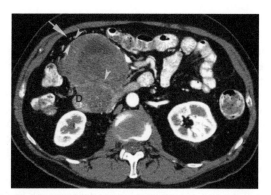

Fig. 1. Primary duodenal GIST. Contrast-enhanced CT scan shows a heterogeneous enhancing, exophytic mass (*arrow*) arising from the second segment of the duodenum (D). Note multiple small tumor vessels (*arrowheads*) within the mass.

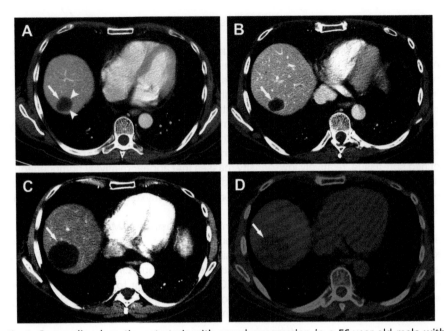

Fig. 2. Responding hepatic metastasis with pseudoprogression in a 56-year-old male with duodenal GIST. (*A*) Pretreatment contrast-enhanced CT showed an enhancing hepatic metastasis (*arrow*) in segment 7 with the tumor density measured 40 HU. Note the peripheral enhancing component (*small arrows*). (*B*) Contrast-enhanced CT image obtained at 2 months after treatment demonstrated a minimal decrease in size of the hepatic metastases (*arrow*) but with a significant decrease in CT density (27 HU). The peripheral enhancement is no longer evident. This is typical of responding GIST. (*C* and *D*) Contrast-enhanced CT image (*C*) obtained at 7 month after treatment showed a homogenously hypoattenuating tumor with a continuous decrease in tumor density (18 HU). Notice the significant increase in tumor size (*arrows*) with no appreciable glucose uptake on the corresponding FDG-PET image. (*D*) Note the fused CT image in the background. The enlarging homogenous tumor with a continuous decrease in tumor density should not be confused with a progressing tumor.

months and may be seen as early as 1 week after treatment (Haesun Choi, MD, unpublished data).

In general, GISTs do decrease in size after targeted therapy, but often it takes several months for the tumors to decrease enough in size to satisfy the traditional size-based response evaluation criteria, such as the Response Evaluation Criteria in Solid Tumors (RECIST),[25] World Health Organization criteria,[26] or Southwest Oncology Group criteria.[27] The median time to evidence of tumor shrinkage on CT is about 3 to 4 months, although it sometimes may take 6 to 12 months or longer.[11–13,18] More importantly, it should be noted that responding GISTs sometimes increase in size because of intratumoral hemorrhage, necrosis, or myxoid degeneration.[28] In these cases, observation of changes in tumor density (indicating a decrease in density) and in the enhancement pattern (indicating a decrease in tumor vasculature) aid to reaching the correct conclusion (see **Fig. 2**).

While traditional size-based criteria underestimate the responses of GIST to targeted therapy,[11–13,18,20,29–31] the use of new imaging modalities, such as PET[11,18,30,32,33] or perfusion CT,[21] and new CT-response evaluation criteria[29,31,34] have been advocated. Choi and colleagues[31] reported that a 10% decrease in the sum of the unidimensional

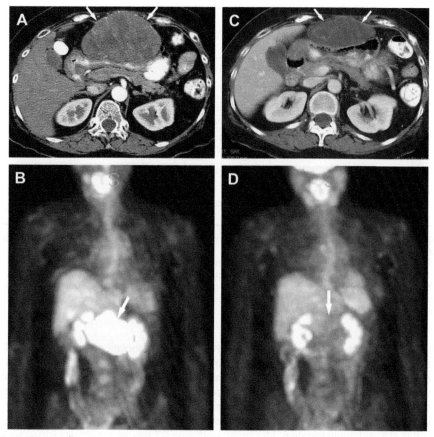

Fig. 3. Responding gastrointestinal stromal tumor in a 59-year-old woman with recurrent gastric GIST in the omentum. (*A* and *B*) Pretreatment contrast-enhanced CT scan (*A*) shows a large, enhancing omental mass (*arrow*) abutting the anterior surface of the stomach corresponding to the mass (*arrow*) with markedly increased glucose update shown on pretreatment FDG-PET (*B*). (*C* and *D*) Contrast-enhanced CT scan (*C*) obtained 2 months after treatment showed that the mass (*arrow*) has decreased in size and become homogeneous, with a marked decrease in CT density corresponding to the mass (*arrow*) with no appreciable glucose uptake shown on FDG-PET (*D*) obtained at the same time.

tumor size or a 15% decrease in tumor density, as determined by the CT attenuation coefficient in Hounsfield units, at the first follow-up (2 months) following treatment can best separate the good responders and poor responders, and that response at this time is an excellent predictor of progression-free survival. The same investigators proposed modified CT response criteria (**Table 1**) using both tumor density and unidimensional measurement of tumor size,[31] of which reproducibility was confirmed in an extended group of patients.[29] Holdsworth and colleagues[34] reported similar results using the sum of products of bidimensional measurement. The investigators reported that an 8.25% decrease in tumor size at 1 month following treatment best separated the group of patients in whom treatment failed and those in whom it did not. The investigators concluded that stability or any decrease in the sum of products of bidimensional measurement at 1 month following treatment was a strong indicator of

Table 1	
Modified CT response evaluation criteria	
Response	**Definition**
CR	Disappearance of all lesions.
	No new lesions.
PR	A decrease in size[a] of ≥ 10% or a decrease in tumor density (HU) ≥ 15% on CT.
	No new lesions.
	No obvious progression of nonmeasurable disease.
SD	Does not meet the criteria of CR, PR, or PD.
	No symptomatic deterioration attributed to tumor progression.
PD	An increase in tumor size of ≥ 10% and does not meet criteria of PR by tumor density (HU) on CT.
	New lesions.
	New intratumoral nodules or increase in the size of the existing intratumoral nodules.

Abbreviations: CR, complete response; HU, Hounsfield unit; PD, progression of disease; PR, partial response; SD, stable disease.
[a] The Sum of longest diameters of target lesions as defined in RECIST.[25]
From Choi H, Charnsangavej C, Faria SC, et al. Correlation of computed tomography and positron emission tomography in patients with metastatic gastrointestinal stromal tumor treated at a single institution with imatinib mesylate: proposal of new computed tomography response criteria. J Clin Oncol 2007;25(13):1753–9; with permission.

time-to-treatment failure in 52 patients. However, this observation has not been validated yet. Trent and colleagues[21] performed perfusion CT and FDG-PET in GIST patients before and after treatment with imatinib mesylate at 3, 5, or 7 days, and found that PET responders (>30% decrease in standardized uptake value) had decreases in both blood flow and blood volume to tumors, while nonresponders had an increase in blood flow and less increase in blood volume. Use of perfusion CT in response evaluation is still under investigation. Moreover, perfusion CT requires special postprocessing software, careful monitoring of data acquisition and, in particular, careful analysis of the data for reducibility.

Surveillance

Contrast-enhanced CT plays an important role in surveillance and the early detection of tumor recurrence or progression that might signal the clonal emergence of resistance to ongoing targeted treatment.[35,36]

After treatment, tumors become hypodense and their size may gradually decrease and eventually stabilize. Recurrence or disease progression is traditionally diagnosed by finding an increase in tumor size or the development of new lesions at the site of previous disease or by finding distant metastasis. However, as mentioned previously, increased tumor size alone without a change in tumor enhancement or tumor vessels may not accurately represent disease progression. It is also notable that the development of an intratumoral enhancing nodule is often an earliest sign of disease progression. This is observed within a treated hypodense tumor without an increase in tumor size (**Fig. 4**).[36,37] Thorough analysis of each treated lesion is required to identify these new intratumoral nodules. If tumor recurrence or disease progression is suspected, short-term follow-up (eg, 1 month) using well-designed contrast-enhanced CT imaging may be performed for confirmative diagnosis. Whenever the CT findings are inconclusive or inconsistent with clinical findings, FDG-PET is indicated.

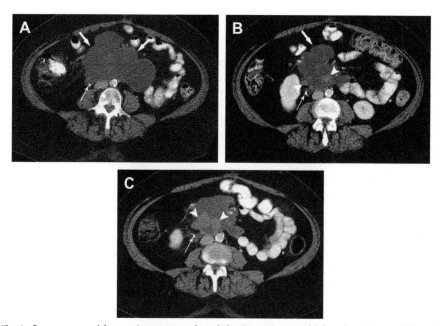

Fig. 4. Recurrence with new intratumoral nodules in a 56 year-old female with small bowel GIST. (*A*) The 7-month posttreatment contrast-enhanced CT showed a treated GIST (*large arrow*) in the mesentery with homogenously decreased density. A right ureteral stent (*small arrow*) was in place. (*B, C*) At 16 months after treatment, the contrast-enhanced CT (*B*) showed a continuous decrease in size of the mass (*large arrow*). Note, however, the new intratumoral enhancing nodules (*arrowheads* in *B* and *C*) that were growing rapidly on the contrast-enhanced CT (*C*) obtained at 22 months. These intratumoral nodules eventually filled in the tumor on further follow-up CTs (not shown).

Technical Limitations

In the management of GISTs, it can be a challenge to properly time the acquisition of biphasic or triphasic contrast-enhanced images. Hypervascular hepatic metastases from GISTs may be missed if the images are acquired only at the portal-venous phase or if a poorly designed multiphasic technique is used. If a well-designed multiphasic technique is unavailable, the acquisition of unenhanced images, in conjunction with conventional enhanced images, can be a good alternative for tumor detection and possibly tumor characterization.[28]

Note should also be made that the tumor density can be increased by intratumoral hemorrhage, which often develops within responding GISTs. This hemorrhage should not be confused with increased enhancement. MRI might be helpful to differentiate hemorrhage from solid tumor if unenhanced CT images are not available.[28]

POSITRON EMISSION TOMOGRAPHY

FDG-PET is a metabolic imaging technique on the basis of regional glucose metabolism at the cellular level. FDG is a glucose analog. Unlike glucose, however, it remains trapped within a cell without being further metabolized after it is phosphorylated. Therefore, malignant cells with increased glycolysis[38,39] and increased glucose uptake will trap FDG within them. Thus, FDG uptake in tumors is thought to represent the regional glucose metabolic rate of viable tumor cells. Over expression of the GLUT-1 glucose transporter is also thought to be responsible for greater accumulation of the FDG in some tumors.

The metabolic activity on FDG-PET can be quantitated by measuring the standardized uptake value (SUV) or by calculating the metabolic rate from dynamic imaging using kinetic analysis. Although quantitative dynamic imaging by kinetic analysis is more accurate than SUV measurement and is independent of imaging time, it has not been used in clinical practice because it is more difficult to perform and is costly.[40] Maximum SUV (SUV_{max}) is most commonly used to determine FDG uptake over a defined time in attenuation-corrected PET images.

Initial Evaluation

FDG-PET is highly sensitive in detecting tumors with high glucose metabolism in the body[41–43] but is nonspecific in making a diagnosis. Thus, the primary role for PET in the initial evaluation of biopsy-proven GISTs is in staging. Baseline FDG-PET is recommended in patients in whom FDG-PET will be used to monitor therapy or who require a very short follow-up (2–3 weeks), such as those with marginally resectable GIST.[10]

In general, for tumors less than 1 cm in size, FDG-PET is not reliable in identifying metabolically active lesions.[44,45] The tumors smaller than 1 cm can be readily detected when there is enough glucose metabolism within the tumor. Use of PET-CT may also allow the detection of smaller lesions. In GIST, it has been reported that the overall sensitivity of FDG-PET is approximately 80% in detection at initial presentation; patients with negative uptake on pretreatment FDG-PET had tumors ranging from 1.0 cm to 4.7 cm.[20] Similarly, Hersh and colleagues[46] found negative results on pretreatment FDG-PET in four out of eight patients. These four patients had homogeneous tumors on CT images, with a mean diameter of 6 cm (range 3 cm–8 cm).

Response Evaluation and Surveillance

FDG-PET has been shown to be highly sensitive and specific in detecting early response and to be useful in predicting long-term response to targeted treatments in patients with metastatic GISTs.[47] FDG-PET response characterized by a marked decrease in glucose metabolism (see **Fig. 3**) can be seen at as early as 24 hours after a single dose of imatinib.[48] Changes of SUV_{max} as absolute values or as percentage changes relative to baseline are used to determine the efficacy of treatment.

Response evaluation using FDG-PET is particularly recommended for those requiring a timely decision for or against surgery, such as those with marginally resectable GISTs or resectable GISTs with a risk of significant morbidity.[10] Knowledge of early response (eg, within 2–3 weeks) in these patients might be beneficial.[10] Likewise, rapid monitoring of therapeutic response by FDG-PET may be needed after adjusting the dose of imatinib.[10] For patients who need or are planned to have early follow-up (within 1 month of treatment initiation) using FDG-PET, a baseline pretreatment FDG-PET may also be needed.

FDG-PET may help to resolve ambiguous findings on CT or MRI. For example, FDG-PET can differentiate between pseudoprogression (see **Fig. 2**), with an increase in size because of myxoid degeneration or intratumoral bleeding, and true tumor progression. In addition, whenever there are inconsistencies between clinical features and CT or MRI findings during the course of the disease, FDG-PET is indicated. As mentioned earlier, short-term follow-up (eg, 1 month after treatment starts) by means of well-designed contrast-enhanced CT is a good alternative in these situations.

Re-emergence of FDG uptake has been reported within the responding GISTs; this effect occurred within days after imatinib was discontinued.[49] This may reflect the cytostatic (as opposed to cytotoxic) activity of this targeted agent and suggests that finding a decrease in uptake or no appreciable uptake on FDG-PET images after treatment may not necessarily reflect tumor viability. In general, it is recommended to keep the patients on a systemic treatment until drug toxicity or significant clinical progression is developed.

Technical Limitations

While FDG-PET has a clear benefit in the clinical management of GIST, there are a few technical imitations of which to be aware.

The FDG uptake is determined by the acquisition technique, the scanner quality control, region-of-interest determination, and the patient's blood glucose level at the time of examination. There is currently no consensus on the best or most appropriate image acquisition technique (eg, time to acquire the images, patient preparation, attenuation correction, and FDG dose) between institutions. Use of a nonoptimized technique will affect the accuracy of FDG uptake measurement, and technical variations between institutions could affect the quantitative response evaluation when SUV is measured. Recognizing the impact of technique on accurate SUV measurement is particularly important in designing multicenter trials. An expert panel of the Cancer Imaging Program of National Cancer Institute has published consensus recommendations for the use of FDG-PET as an indicator of therapeutic response in institute-sponsored trials.[40] The standard protocol (eg, the optimum FDG dose), however, has not yet been determined.

More importantly, there are no standardized PET-response evaluation criteria for GISTs. The European Organization for Research and Treatment of Cancer (EORTC) established guidelines for the use of FDG-PET as a biomarker of response in 1999, defining a 25% reduction in SUV_{max} as the threshold for partial metabolic response.[50] However, this guideline is based on the reproducibility of SUV measurements, not on patient clinical outcome.[50] Studies have shown that using an SUV_{max} cutoff of 2.5 measured at 1 month after targeted therapy correlates with patient outcome.[47,49] Jager and colleagues[19] reported that a decrease in SUV_{max} by 65% at 1 week after treatment indicated good response. Choi and colleagues[31] have shown that a combination of percentage changes and absolute values of SUV_{max} measurement at 2 months after treatment (decrease by a more than 70% decrease in SUV_{max} or to an absolute value of SUV_{max} of less than 2.5) was an excellent prognostic indicator. Recently, Holdsworth and colleagues[51] reported that using an SUV_{max} of 3.4 and a 40% reduction in SUV_{max} could predict the time to treatment failure better than using the 2.5 SUV_{max} threshold and 25% reduction in SUV_{max} recommended by the EORTC.

Finally, static FDG uptake alone sometimes may not be able to differentiate between malignant and benign lesions with increased FDG uptake: for example, infection, inflammation, and posttreatment changes. Careful analysis of the corresponding CT images in such cases is therefore essential.

ULTRASOUND

Endoscopic ultrasonography (EUS) may be used in evaluating small (<2 cm) GISTs that are incidentally found during endoscopy. The high-frequency probe (12 mHz–20 mHz) used in EUS can delineate each layer of bowel wall and, therefore, may reliably locate tumor origin within or outside of the wall. EUS also can evaluate the tumor vascularity when used in conjunction with Doppler ultrasonography. EUS is most useful in the esophagus, stomach, duodenum, and anorectum. EUS is, however, not a routine imaging modality because of its limited penetration and field of view. Thus, CT should always be performed to accurately estimate the extent of disease.[52,53]

Although transabdominal ultrasonography may, in an expert's hand, be used to evaluate hepatic metastasis, this technique is inappropriate for evaluating the peritoneal cavity or large tumors in staging or monitoring the disease following treatment.

Ultrasound can be an excellent tool guiding the biopsy procedure, however. A core biopsy using a large-bore needle (16G) is required for proper sampling in GIST. A concern of insufficient sampling using needle aspiration has been reported.[54,55]

MAGNETIC RESONANCE IMAGING

MRI is superior to contrast-enhanced CT in evaluating the hepatic metastasis and rectal GIST with superior soft-tissue contrast and direct multiplanar acquisition capability. However, MRI is not the primary imaging modality of choice in evaluating GIST patients because of its general limited sensitivity in detecting peritoneal tumors. However, thorough analysis of well-designed, dedicated MRI (thin-section, such as <5 mm, fat-saturated T1-weighed images), can provide good visualization of the peritoneal cavity in most patients.

On MRI, GISTs are generally well defined; the solid portions of the masses are typically of low- to intermediate-signal intensity on T1-weighted images and high signal intensity on T2-weighted images. As in CT, the tumors enhance after administration of an intravenous contrast agent.[56] Intravenous contrast helps to delineate viable solid components and nonenhanced necrotic areas. Internal hemorrhage may have signal intensity varying from high to low on both T1- and T2-weighted images, depending on the age.[57] MRI can be used to differentiate the possible high-density intratumoral mass shown on CT images from hemorrhage. Dynamic contrast-enhanced MRI can be used to evaluate tumor viability and to quantitate the status of angiogenesis. However, to the authors' knowledge, no published series has evaluated the value of this imaging technique in management of GISTs.

Table 2
CT and FDG-PET in management of gastrointestinal stromal tumors

	CT	FDG-PET
Primary role	Imaging modality of choice 1. Diagnosis 2. Staging 3. Response evaluation 4. Surveillance	1. Problem solving 2. Short term follow-up for marginally resectable GIST
Information	Anatomy and tumor vascularity	Regional glucose metabolism
Quantitation	1. Degree of contrast enhancement (Hounsfield unit) 2. Size	Glucose metabolism (SUV)
Limitation	1. No technical limitation—widely accepted 2. Underestimation of response using a standard size-based criteria[a]	1. No standard image acquisition technique 2. No standard criteria for response evaluation 3. Costly, limited in availability

[a] RECIST, World Health Organization criteria, Southwest Oncology Group criteria: A combination of contrast enhancement and size change provides response information with high confidence.

SUMMARY

The emergence of new molecularly targeted agents, the tyrosine receptor blockers, has revolutionized not only clinical outcomes of patients but also the radiologic assessment of treatment response and surveillance.

CT is available worldwide and is highly efficient with good technical reproducibility. CT is the imaging modality of choice for the initial evaluation, staging, and monitoring of treatment response in GIST. Although traditional size-based response criteria, such as RECIST, have been shown to be inappropriate in evaluating GIST responses to targeted therapy, new CT criteria using modified size criteria and unique CT features (eg, change in tumor density) have been proposed with promising results. FDG-PET is highly sensitive and specific in response evaluation of GISTs to systemic treatment and is indicated when there are inconsistencies between CT and clinical findings or inconclusive CT images. A short-term (1 month) follow-up CT can be a good alternative in these patients. Role of ultrasound is primarily in guiding a biopsy. MRI can also useful in characterizing the hepatic lesions, rectal GIST, and in those who are contraindicated for contrast enhanced CT. MRI should be carefully designed and analyzed for possible peritoneal disease. The features of CT and FDG-PET are summarized in **Table 2**.

REFERENCES

1. Miettinen M, Lasota J. Gastrointestinal stromal tumors (GISTs): definition, occurrence, pathology, differential diagnosis and molecular genetics. Pol J Pathol 2003;54(1):3–24.
2. DeMatteo RP, Lewis JJ, Leung D, et al. Two hundred gastrointestinal stromal tumors: recurrence patterns and prognostic factors for survival. Ann Surg 2000; 231(1):51–8.
3. Gold JS, Dematteo RP. Combined surgical and molecular therapy: the gastrointestinal stromal tumor model. Ann Surg 2006;244(2):176–84.
4. Langer C, Gunawan B, Schuler P, et al. Prognostic factors influencing surgical management and outcome of gastrointestinal stromal tumours. Br J Surg 2003; 90(3):332–9.
5. Mazur MT, Clark HB. Gastric stromal tumors. Reappraisal of histogenesis. Am J Surg Pathol 1983;7(6):507–19.
6. Nishida T, Hirota S. Biological and clinical review of stromal tumors in the gastrointestinal tract. Histol Histopathol 2000;15(4):1293–301.
7. Hirota S, Isozaki K, Moriyama Y, et al. Gain-of-function mutations of c-kit in human gastrointestinal stromal tumors. Science 1998;279(5350):577–80.
8. DeMatteo RP. The GIST of targeted cancer therapy: a tumor (gastrointestinal stromal tumor), a mutated gene (c-kit), and a molecular inhibitor (STI571). Ann Surg Oncol 2002;9(9):831–9.
9. Heinrich MC, Corless CL, Duensing A, et al. PDGFRA activating mutations in gastrointestinal stromal tumors. Science 2003;299(5607):708–10.
10. Demetri GD, Benjamin RS, Blanke CD, et al. NCCN Task Force report: management of patients with gastrointestinal stromal tumor (GIST)–update of the NCCN clinical practice guidelines. J Natl Compr Canc Netw 2007;2(Suppl 5):S1–29.
11. Demetri GD, von Mehren M, Blanke CD, et al. Efficacy and safety of imatinib mesylate in advanced gastrointestinal stromal tumors. N Engl J Med 2002;347(7): 472–80.

12. Joensuu H, Roberts PJ, Sarlomo-Rikala M, et al. Effect of the tyrosine kinase inhibitor STI571 in a patient with a metastatic gastrointestinal stromal tumor. N Engl J Med 2001;344(14):1052–6.

13. van Oosterom AT, Judson I, Verweij J, et al. Safety and efficacy of imatinib (STI571) in metastatic gastrointestinal stromal tumours: a phase I study. Lancet 2001;358(9291):1421–3.

14. Blanke C, Joensuu G, Demetri M, et al. Long-term follow up of advanced gastrointestinal stromal tumor (GIST) patients treated with imatinib mesylate [abstract 2]. In: Proceedings of the 2004 Gastrointestinal Cancers Symposium: current status and future directions for prevention and management. American Society of Clinical Oncology, Alexandria: 2004;43.

15. Verweij J, Casali PG, Zalcberg J, et al. Progression-free survival in gastrointestinal stromal tumours with high-dose imatinib: randomised trial. Lancet 2004; 364(9440):1127–34.

16. Demetri GD, van Oosterom AT, Garrett CR, et al. Efficacy and safety of sunitinib in patients with advanced gastrointestinal stromal tumour after failure of imatinib: a randomised controlled trial. Lancet 2006;368(9544):1329–38.

17. Demetri GD, Benjamin RS, Blanke CD, et al. NCCN Task Force report: optimal management of patients with gastrointestinal stromal tumors (gist)-expansion and update of NCCN clinical practice guidelines. J Natl Compr Canc Netw 2004;2(Suppl 1):S1–26.

18. Stroobants S, Goeminne J, Seegers M, et al. 18FDG-Positron emission tomography for the early prediction of response in advanced soft tissue sarcoma treated with imatinib mesylate (Glivec). Eur J Cancer 2003;39(14): 2012–20.

19. Jager PL, Gietema JA, van der Graaf WT. Imatinib mesylate for the treatment of gastrointestinal stromal tumours: best monitored with FDG PET. Nucl Med Commun 2004;25(5):433–8.

20. Choi H, Charnsangavej C, de Castro Faria S, et al. CT evaluation of the response of gastrointestinal stromal tumors after imatinib mesylate treatment: a quantitative analysis correlated with FDG PET findings. AJR Am J Roentgenol 2004;183(6): 1619–28.

21. Trent JC, Choi H, Hunt H, et al. Apoptotic and anti-vascular activity of imatinib in GIST patients [abstract 9001]. In: Proceedings of the 42nd annual meeting of American Society of Clinical Oncology, Orlando: 2005.

22. Berger F, Schlemmer M, Saam T, et al. Initial experiences utilizing perfusion CT in the follow-up of patients with gastrointestinal stromal tumors under imatinib mesylate treatment [abstract SSM09-05]. In: Programs and abstracts of 93th Scientific Assembly and Annual Meeting of Radiological Society of North America, Chicago: 2007. p. 534.

23. Lee TY. Functional CT: physiological models. Trends Biotechnol 2002;20:S3–10.

24. Nilsson B, Bumming P, Meis-Kindblom JM, et al. Gastrointestinal stromal tumors: the incidence, prevalence, clinical course, and prognostication in the preimatinib mesylate era—a population-based study in western Sweden. Cancer 2005; 103(4):821–9.

25. Therasse P, Arbuck SG, Eisenhauer EA, et al. New guidelines to evaluate the response to treatment in solid tumors. European Organization for Research and Treatment of Cancer, National Cancer Institute of the United States, National Cancer Institute of Canada. J Natl Cancer Inst 2000;92(3):205–16.

26. Miller AB, Hoogstraten B, Staquet M, et al. Reporting results of cancer treatment. Cancer 1981;47(1):207–14.

27. Green S, Weiss GR. Southwest Oncology Group standard response criteria, endpoint definitions and toxicity criteria. Invest New Drugs 1992;10(4):239–53.
28. Hong X, Choi H, Loyer EM, et al. Gastrointestinal stromal tumor: role of CT in diagnosis and in response evaluation and surveillance after treatment with imatinib. Radiographics 2006;26(2):481–95.
29. Benjamin RS, Choi H, Macapinlac HA, et al. We should desist using RECIST, at least in GIST. J Clin Oncol 2007;25(13):1760–4.
30. Antoch G, Kanja J, Bauer S, et al. Comparison of PET, CT, and dual-modality PET/CT imaging for monitoring of imatinib (STI571) therapy in patients with gastrointestinal stromal tumors. J Nucl Med 2004;45(3):357–65.
31. Choi H, Charnsangavej C, Faria SC, et al. Correlation of computed tomography and positron emission tomography in patients with metastatic gastrointestinal stromal tumor treated at a single institution with imatinib mesylate: proposal of new computed tomography response criteria. J Clin Oncol 2007;25(13):1753–9.
32. Van den Abbeele AD, Badawi RD. Use of positron emission tomography in oncology and its potential role to assess response to imatinib mesylate therapy in gastrointestinal stromal tumors (GISTs). Eur J Cancer 2002;38(Suppl 5):S60–5.
33. Reddy MP, Reddy P, Lilien DL. F-18 FDG PET imaging in gastrointestinal stromal tumor. Clin Nucl Med 2003;28(8):677–9.
34. Holdsworth CH, Manola J, Badawi RD, et al. Use of computerized tomography (CT) as an early prognostic indicator of response to imatinib mesylate (IM) in pateints with gastrointestinal stromal tumors (GIST) [abstrast 3011]. In: Proceedings of the American Society of Clinical Oncology Annual meeting. New Orleans, Louisiana, June 5–8, 2004.
35. Chen LL, Trent JC, Wu EF, et al. A missense mutation in KIT kinase domain 1 correlates with imatinib resistance in gastrointestinal stromal tumors. Cancer Res 2004;64(17):5913–9.
36. Desai J, Shankar S, Heinrich MC, et al. Clonal evolution of resistance to imatinib in patients with metastatic gastrointestinal stromal tumors. Clin Cancer Res 2007;13(18 Pt 1):5398–405.
37. Choi H. Response evaluation of gastrointestinal stromal tumors. Oncologist 2008;13(Suppl 2):4–7.
38. Weber G. Enzymology of cancer cells (first of two parts). N Engl J Med 1977;296(9):486–92.
39. Weber G. Enzymology of cancer cells (second of two parts). N Engl J Med 1977;296(10):541–51.
40. Shankar LK, Hoffman JM, Bacharach S, et al. Consensus recommendations for the use of 18F-FDG PET as an indicator of therapeutic response in patients in National Cancer Institute Trials. J Nucl Med 2006;47(6):1059–66.
41. Delbeke D. Oncological applications of FDG PET imaging. J Nucl Med 1999;40(10):1706–15.
42. Marsden P, Sutcliffe-Goulden J. Principles and technology of PET scanning. Nucl Med Commun 2000;21(3):221–4.
43. Stokkel MP, Draisma A, Pauwels EK. Positron emission tomography with 2-[18F]-fluoro-2-deoxy-D-glucose in oncology. Part IIIb: therapy response monitoring in colorectal and lung tumours, head and neck cancer, hepatocellular carcinoma and sarcoma. J Cancer Res Clin Oncol 2001;127(5):278–85.
44. Kelloff GJ, Sullivan DM, Wilson W, et al. FDG-PET lymphoma demonstration project invitational workshop. Acad Radiol 2007;14(3):330–9.

45. Ung YC, Maziak DE, Vanderveen JA, et al. 18Fluorodeoxyglucose positron emission tomography in the diagnosis and staging of lung cancer: a systematic review. J Natl Cancer Inst 2007;99(23):1753–67.
46. Hersh MR, Choi J, Garrett C, et al. Imaging gastrointestinal stromal tumors. Cancer Control 2005;12(2):111–5.
47. Van den Abbeele AD, BR, Cliche J, et al. 18F-FDG-PET predicts response to imatinib mesylate (Gleevec) in patients with advanced gastrointestinal stromal tumors (GIST) [abstract 1610]. In: Proceedings of the 38th Annual Meeting of the American Society of Clinical Oncology, Orlando; 2002. p. 403a.
48. Van den Abbeele AD for the GIST Collaborative PET Study Group Dana Farber Cancer Institute, Boston, Massachusetts; OHSU, Portland, Oregon. Helsinki University Central Hospital, Turku University Central Hospital, Finland, Novartis Oncology.F18-FDG-PET provides early evidence of biological response to STI57 in patients with malignant gastrointestinal stromal tumors (GIST) [abstract 1444]. In: Proceedings of the 37th Annual Meeting of the American Society of Clinical Oncology, San Francisco; 2001. p. 362a.
49. Van den Abbeele AD, Badawi RD, Manola J, et al. Effects of cessation of imatinib mesylate (IM) therapy in patients (pts) with IM-refractory gastrointestinal stromal tumors (GIST) as visualized by FDG-PET scanning. J Clin Oncol 2004; 22(Suppl 14):198.
50. Young H, Baum R, Cremerius U, et al. Measurement of clinical and subclinical tumour response using [18F]-fluorodeoxyglucose and positron emission tomography: review and 1999 EORTC recommendations. European Organization for Research and Treatment of Cancer (EORTC) PET Study Group. Eur J Cancer 1999;35(13):1773–82.
51. Holdsworth CH, Badawi RD, Manola JB, et al. CT and PET: early prognostic indicators of response to imatinib mesylate in patients with gastrointestinal stromal tumor. AJR Am J Roentgenol 2007;189(6):W324–30.
52. Buscarini E, Stasi MD, Rossi S, et al. Endosonographic diagnosis of submucosal upper gastrointestinal tract lesions and large fold gastropathies by catheter ultrasound probe. Gastrointest Endosc 1999;49(2):184–91.
53. Layke JC, Lopez PP. Gastric cancer: diagnosis and treatment options. Am Fam Physician 2004;69(5):1133–40.
54. Kimura H, Shima Y, Kinoshita S, et al. Endosonographic misdiagnosis of tumor recurrence after surgery for malignant GIST. Endoscopy 2002;34(3):238.
55. Fu K, Eloubeidi MA, Jhala NC, et al. Diagnosis of gastrointestinal stromal tumor by endoscopic ultrasound-guided fine needle aspiration biopsy—a potential pitfall. Ann Diagn Pathol 2002;6(5):294–301.
56. Levy AD, Remotti HE, Thompson WM, et al. Gastrointestinal stromal tumors: radiologic features with pathologic correlation. Radiographics 2003;23(2): 283–304.
57. Hasegawa S, Semelka RC, Noone TC, et al. Gastric stromal sarcomas: correlation of MR imaging and histopathologic findings in nine patients. Radiology 1998; 208(3):591–5.

Contemporary Pathology of Gastrointestinal Stromal Tumors

Bernadette Liegl, MD[a,b], Jason L. Hornick, MD, PhD[b],
Alexander J.F. Lazar, MD, PhD[c],*

KEYWORDS

- Gastrointestinal stromal tumor • KIT • Pathology
- Risk assessment • Molecular prognosis • Targeted therapy
- Biomarkers • Post-treatment changes

Until recently, a large group of mesenchymal tumors arising in the gastrointestinal (GI) tract have been classified as smooth muscle tumors or occasionally as neural tumors.[1] The term "stromal tumors" was introduced in 1983 by Mazur and Clark[2] but was not widely adopted until the early 1990s, when it was discovered that most stromal tumors arising in the GI tract are reactive for CD34,[3] the first relatively specific marker for gastrointestinal stromal tumors (GISTs). During the 1990s, several groups noted similarities between GIST cells and the interstitial cells of Cajal,[4–7] a group of cells located in the muscularis propria and around the myenteric plexus throughout the GI tract, serving as pacemakers for peristaltic contractions.[8,9] Studies at that time revealed that Cajal cells express the receptor tyrosine kinase (RTK) KIT and are developmentally dependent on its ligand, stem cell factor.[8] In 1998, Hirota and colleagues[5] reported activating mutations in the *KIT* gene in GIST, as well as expression of the KIT protein by immunohistochemistry, and in 2003 Heinrich and colleagues[10] found that a subset of GISTs lacking *KIT* mutations can harbor mutations in the homologous RTK gene platelet-derived growth factor receptor α (*PDGFRA*). In total, 85% to 90% of GISTs harbor activating mutations in either *KIT* or *PDGFRA*,[10,11] and the resultant

This work supported in part by the University of Texas M.D. Anderson Cancer Center Physician Scientist Program (A.J.L.). B.L. was supported by the FWF Austrian Science Fund.

[a] Department of Pathology, Medical University of Graz, Auenbruggerplatz 25, A 8036 Graz, Austria

[b] Department of Pathology, Brigham and Women's Hospital and Harvard Medical School, 75 Francis Street, Boston, MA 02115, USA

[c] Department of Pathology, Sarcoma Research Center, The University of Texas M.D. Anderson Cancer Center, 1515 Holcombe Blvd—Unit 85, Houston, TX, USA

* Corresponding author.

E-mail address: alazar@mdanderson.org (A.J.F. Lazar).

constitutively activated oncoproteins serve as crucial diagnostic and therapeutic targets in GIST.[10,11] These findings were confirmed and expanded by several other laboratories, which led to a rapid evolution in the understanding of the biology of these tumors and the development of molecular targeted treatment of GISTs. Within the past decade, GISTs, formerly viewed as among the most treatment-refractory sarcomas, with fewer than 10% of patients showing clinical response to conventional chemotherapies or radiation therapy,[12,13] are now regarded as highly treatable with the tyrosine kinase inhibitors (TKIs) imatinib mesylate and sunitinib malate, with additional alternative targeted agents now in clinical trials. GISTs are an important paradigm of molecular targeted therapy in solid tumors. Optimal application of treatment, however, demands accurate tumor classification and risk assessment. These critical subjects are addressed in this article.

EPIDEMIOLOGY

The incidence of GIST in the United States and Europe is difficult to determine because GISTs have been recognized and uniformly diagnosed as a discrete entity only since the late 1990s. Recent population-based studies in some European countries found an incidence between 11 and 14.5 cases per million.[14–16] These findings would translate into an annual incidence in the United States of 4,000 to 5,000 cases. However, the prevalence of GIST may be even higher, as many patients live with the disease for years, or develop very small GISTs only detected incidentally at the time of autopsy or when a gastrectomy is performed for another reason.[17–19] Irrespective of tumor size, GISTs share morphologic features and immunoreactivity for KIT and often contain an oncogenic mutation in the *KIT* or *PDGFRA* gene,[17,18,20,21] indicating that not all small GISTs progress rapidly into large tumors, despite the presence of RTK gene mutations.

CLINICAL AND PATHOLOGIC FEATURES
Clinical Features

The majority of patients diagnosed with GISTs are between 40 and 80 years of age (median age approximately 60 years).[22] There is no clear sex predilection. Rarely, GISTs occur in children; pediatric GISTs are considered a separate clinicopathologic entity, occurring predominantly in the second decade.[23,24] Most GISTs are sporadic, but familial GISTs associated with inherited germline mutations have been identified.[25–31] GISTs have also been demonstrated in association with syndromes such as neurofibromatosis type I,[32–34] Carney triad (gastric GIST, paraganglioma, pulmonary chondroma),[35,36] and the Carney-Stratakis "dyad" (paraganglioma, gastric GIST).[37] Both hereditary GIST syndromes and pediatric GISTs are discussed separately in other articles of this issue of *Clinics*.

GISTs occur throughout the GI tract from the esophagus to the anus. The most common sites are the stomach (60%) and jejunum and ileum (30%). GISTs less commonly affect the duodenum (5%), colorectum (4%), and esophagus or appendix (<1%).[22,38–40] Tumors lacking any association with the bowel wall have been referred to as extra-gastrointestinal stromal tumors (termed EGISTs) and occur in the omentum, mesentery, or retroperitoneum.[41,42] Approximately 70% of GISTs present with clinical symptoms, whereas 20% are asymptomatic and 10% are incidentally detected at autopsy.[15] The median tumor size from these three categories is 8.9 cm, 2.7 cm, and 3.4 cm, respectively.[15] Patients with clinically malignant GISTs may present with disseminated disease. Metastases occur primarily in the liver and abdominal cavity. Metastases to the lung, bone, lymph nodes (with the exception of pediatric

GISTs), skin, or soft tissues are rare and generally only seen in the setting of very late stage disease.[38] While most metastases occur within 5 years of initial surgical resection, metastases can be seen up to 20 years after initial surgery, and thus long-term follow-up of these patients is mandatory.

Macroscopic Features

GISTs present as well circumscribed, highly vascular tumors in the wall or subserosa of the stomach or the intestine. On gross examination, these tumors appear fleshy, pink or tan-white, and may show hemorrhage (**Fig. 1**). Large tumors frequently show cystic degeneration or necrosis even in the absence of prior treatment.

Microscopic Features

Histologically, GISTs can be divided into three different histologic subgroups. Spindle cell GISTs (approximately 70%) are composed of cells with palely eosinophilic, fibrillary cytoplasm, ovoid uniform nuclei, and ill-defined cell borders, often with a somewhat syncytial appearance, arranged in short fascicles or whorls (**Fig. 2A**). Epithelioid GISTs (approximately 20%) are composed of rounded cells with eosinophilic to clear cytoplasm arranged in sheets and nests (**Fig. 2B**). The final group shows mixed spindle cell and epithelioid cytomorphology (approximately 10%).

All these subtypes can vary in cellularity, and the stroma can be sclerotic, collagenous, or myxoid; rarely, calcification may be seen. GISTs located in the small bowel may show distinctive round, elongated, or ovoid aggregates of extracellular collagen bundles, referred to as skeinoid fibers (**Fig. 3A**). GISTs with prominent nuclear palisading (**Fig. 3B**) may mimic a neural tumor, and paranuclear vacuolization (**Fig. 3C**) may be seen in gastric tumors. The significance of these features is not clear. Spindle cell GISTs can also show a storiform growth pattern. In epithelioid GISTs with clear cytoplasm, the tumor cells often show sharp cell borders (see **Fig. 2B**). Tumors with high mitotic activity can be seen in every subgroup. Although GISTs are generally cytologically uniform and monotonous tumors, nuclear atypia can occasionally be pronounced (in approximately 2% of tumors), mimicking a high grade pleomorphic sarcoma (pleomorphic GISTs) (**Fig. 3D**),[43] and rare GISTs showing dedifferentiation, defined as an abrupt transition between a conventional GIST and a KIT-negative anaplastic high-grade sarcoma, have been reported to occur (**Fig. 3 E and F**).[44]

GISTs are increasingly being resected following TKI therapy.[12] GISTs treated with TKIs may show a dramatic decrease in tumor cellularity and stromal changes,

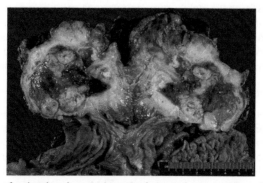

Fig. 1. Gross image of a duodenal gastrointestinal stromal tumor. When this tumor failed to respond to imatinib mesylate, a Whipple resection was required.

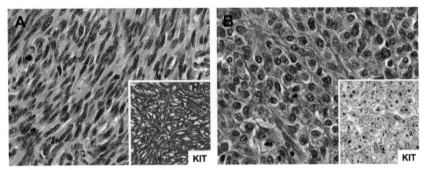

Fig. 2. Major morphologic variants of GIST. (*A*) Spindle cell (400×) and (*B*) epithelioid (400×). The insets show diffuse and dot-like KIT immunoreactivity, respectively (200×).

including marked sclerosis, fibrohyalinosis, or prominent myxoid or pseudochondroid changes (**Fig. 4** A and B). However, viable tumor cells are found in the vast majority of tumor specimens resected after treatment, even if the tumor responded well to therapy (see **Fig. 4** A and B). The tumor cell morphology in treated tumors usually remains similar to the primary tumor, though the cells often appear atrophic with depleted cytoplasm. Occasionally, treatment with TKIs can dramatically alter the morphologic appearance. At the time of tumor progression on TKI, morphologic changes from spindle cell to purely epithelioid cytology (**Fig. 4**C), a pseudopapillary epithelioid appearance,[45] as well as heterologous rhabdomyosarcomatous differentiation (**Fig. 4**D)[46] have been reported. These findings can cause major diagnostic problems, especially when the tumor shows unusual morphology and loses KIT expression. Under these circumstances, mutational analysis can be helpful, as these tumors have been shown to retain their primary *KIT* mutation.[45,46] Pathologists should be aware that unusual morphologic changes can occur, especially in the setting of metastatic, progressing GISTs treated with TKI. With emerging treatment strategies and the use of several different TKIs or other drugs, drug-resistant tumor clones with unusual morphologic features may develop.

Gastrointestinal Stromal Tumors and Neurofibromatosis Type I

Although hereditary syndromes in GISTs and pediatric GISTs will be discussed separately in this issue, the morphologic features of these GISTs are briefly described here. Patients with neurofibromatosis type I (NF1) can have multiple small GISTs in the small bowel. These GISTs show mainly pure spindle cell morphology and are mitotically inactive. These tumors strongly express KIT but are almost universally negative for *KIT* and *PDGFRA* mutations.[32–34,47] Rarely, cases of clinically malignant GISTs in addition to multiple benign tumor nodules have been described in patients with NF1,[40] and their morphologic features are usually similar to sporadic GIST.

Pediatric Gastrointestinal Stromal Tumors

Pediatric GISTs present predominantly in the second decade of life and account for 1% to 2% of all GISTs. Pediatric GISTs show a marked female predominance, are nearly exclusive to the stomach, and show multinodular growth and mainly epithelioid morphology. Although these tumors show KIT expression by immunohistochemistry, only approximately 10% harbor a *KIT* or *PDGFRA* mutation.[23,24] Unlike adult GISTs, these tumors frequently involve lymph nodes.[23] More work is needed to understand the unique pathogenesis of this GIST subset. In young patients diagnosed with

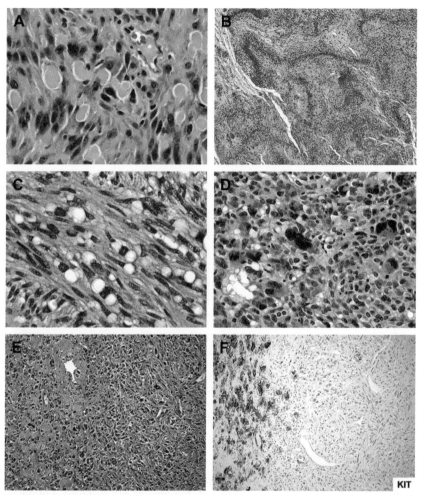

Fig. 3. Other features encountered in GIST. (A) Skeinoid fibers (400×); (B) nuclear palisading (40×); (C) paranuclear vacuolization (400×); (D) cellular pleomorphism (400×); (E) dedifferentiated GIST showing transition from conventional epithelioid morphology (*left*) to an undifferentiated pleomorphic sarcoma (*right*). The conventional component shows diffuse staining for KIT (*left*), whereas the dedifferentiated component is KIT negative (F).

GIST, the presence of one or more lung nodules should raise the possibility of Carney triad presenting with a GIST and pulmonary chondroma.[35,36]

IMMUNOHISTOCHEMICAL MARKERS AND PCR-BASED ASSAYS IN THE DIAGNOSIS OF GASTROINTESTINAL STROMAL TUMORS

KIT has been demonstrated as a very specific and sensitive marker in the differential diagnosis of mesenchymal tumors in the GI tract;[48] around 95% of GISTs express KIT.[5,6,49,50] Different KIT staining patterns can be seen. Most GISTs show strong and diffuse cytoplasmic staining, whereas nearly half show concurrent dot-like (Golgi-pattern) staining (**Fig. 5** A and B). In a minority of cases, a purely dot-like (see

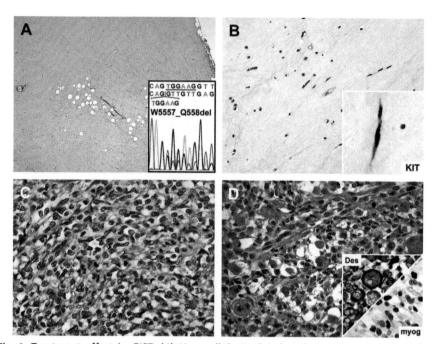

Fig. 4. Treatment effect in GIST. (*A*) Hypocellularity (20×) with inset showing the initial mutation is present and can be detected by polymerase chain reaction (PCR)-based methods; (*B*) higher power with hypocellularity consisting of atrophic spindle cells in a sclerotic stroma (200×) that retain KIT immunoreactivity (inset, 400×); (*C*) acquired resistance to imatinib mesylate can be associated with transformation to epithelioid morphology (400×); (*D*) rhabdomyosarcomatous differentiation is encountered on occasion with TKI resistance (400×), confirmed by cytoplasmic desmin and nuclear myogenin immunoreactivity (*inset*, 400×).

Fig. 2B) or even a membranous staining pattern can be observed. The extent and patterns of KIT staining do not correlate with the type of *KIT* mutation and have no impact on the likelihood of response to imatinib. GISTs showing weak or focal KIT expression and those GISTs completely negative for KIT are more likely to harbor *PDGFRA* mutations and to be wild-type for *KIT* (**Fig. 5**C and D).[51,52] Immunohisto-chemically KIT-negative GISTs account for 4% to 5% of cases[51,52] and preferentially occur in the stomach and omentum, where they often show a pure epithelioid or mixed (spindle cell and epithelioid) cytomorphology. KIT-negative GISTs can cause diagnostic difficulties, but given the rather limited choice in mesenchymal diagnostic considerations at these sites, they can often be diagnosed by excluding other potential mimics by immunohistochemical characterization.

Additional markers commonly expressed in GISTs, although less sensitive and specific than KIT, are CD34, h-caldesmon, and smooth muscle actin (SMA). CD34 is expressed in approximately 80% of gastric, 50% of small intestinal, and approximately 95% of esophageal and rectal GISTs (70% on average),[22,40] whereas h-caldesmon is expressed in more than two-thirds of GISTs[41,53] and SMA in approximately 30%. Expression of SMA has been proposed to be a statistically significant favorable prognostic factor in gastric and small intestinal GISTs,[22,40] but does not appear to be significant in multivariate analysis with other relevant factors. S-100 protein (5%) and

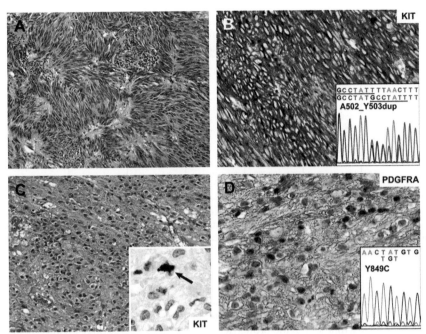

Fig. 5. GIST with mutational events. (*A*) Small bowel GIST (100×); (*B*) KIT immunohistochemistry (200×), inset with exon 9 duplication; (*C*) epithelioid gastric GIST (200×) lacking immunoreactivity for KIT in tumor cells and a single mast cell (*arrow*) serving as an internal positive control (inset, 400×). (*D*) Immunohistochemistry showed diffuse reactivity for PDGFRα (400×) and a point mutation in exon 18 of *PDGFRA* with loss of heterozygosity (*inset*).

cytokeratins (< 1%) are rarely expressed. Desmin expression is uncommon in GISTs (2%); however, in the authors' experience, approximately one-third of KIT-negative GISTs, especially those showing epithelioid morphology and located in the stomach, are desmin positive (see **Fig. 5C**).[54] The most common immunohistochemical profile for GIST with rough percentage reactivities is illustrated in **Fig. 6**. In this context, it should be noted that KIT negativity by no means justifies denying patients therapy with TKIs (imatinib and sunitinib), as a subset of wild-type GISTs and some *PDGFRA*-mutant tumors respond to such treatment.[11,55,56]

Over the last several years, alternative antibodies have emerged for the diagnosis of GIST. These immunomarkers were mainly identified through molecular studies and are of particular interest in the subgroup of KIT-negative GISTs, and those showing only weak or focal KIT expression.

Two recent studies have suggested that antibodies against DOG1 (Discovered On GIST) have greater sensitivity and specificity than KIT and CD34, and that these antibodies could serve as immunohistochemical markers for GIST irrespective of the type of underlying RTK mutation or the presence of KIT expression.[57,58] DOG1 encodes a protein of unknown function that has been shown to be up-regulated by gene-expression profiling. A rabbit polyclonal antibody and recently two mouse monoclonal antibodies against DOG1 (DOG1.1 and DOG1.3), effective in paraffin-embedded tissue, were reported to be superior in sensitivity and specificity to KIT and CD34.[57,58] In the authors' experience, DOG1.1 is a highly sensitive marker for GIST

H&E	CD117 (KIT)	CD34	Smooth muscle actin	S100 protein	Desmin	Pan-keratin
	95%	70%	30%	5%	2%	<1%
+	+	+	+	+	+	+	+	+	+	+	+	+

Fig. 6. The most common immunohistochemical pattern for GIST is diffuse reactivity for KIT (CD117) and CD34. SMA can be reactive, but desmin, S-100 protein and pan-cytokeratin are usually uniformly negative (1×). Percentages of immunoreactivity for each of these markers are listed above.

that is expressed in *KIT*-mutated GISTs and unusual subtypes of GISTs lacking RTK mutations (**Fig. 7**). However, the authors have found that KIT-negative GISTs express DOG1.1 in only 36% of cases, limiting its use in this setting.[54]

PKC-theta is a member of the protein kinase C family that is expressed in virtually all GISTs. Immunohistochemical staining for PKC-theta is positive in GIST, but in the authors' experience, the commercially available antibodies to this protein show significant background staining that limits their clinical utility.[59,60] Furthermore, expression of PKC-theta by immunohistochemistry has been recently demonstrated in leiomyomas, leiomyosarcomas, schwannomas, and desmoid tumors, a finding that questions the diagnostic utility of this marker in GIST.[61]

PDGFRA is a RTK closely related to KIT. Antibodies to this kinase have been proposed to be of use in the identification of KIT-negative GISTs haboring a *PDGFRA* mutation.[62–65] However, PDGFRA is also expressed in other mesenchymal tumors, and the commercially available antibodies do not show reproducible immunohistochemical results in paraffin sections in the experience of every laboratory. Nonetheless, intense staining with this antibody is often seen in gastric epithelioid GISTs that are negative for KIT (see **Fig. 5** C and D), and it can be helpful in this setting,

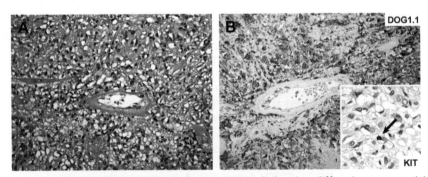

Fig. 7. Novel GIST biomarker. (A) Epithelioid GIST (200×) showing diffuse immunoreactivity for DOG1.1 (B) (200×), whereas KIT is negative with a mast cell serving as an internal positive control (*arrow; inset*) (400×).

though its applicability in spindle cell and mixed GISTs at other sites can be more problematic.

Overall, DOG1.1 seems to be the most promising new marker in addition to KIT, and will likely be diagnostically helpful in at least a subset of KIT-negative tumors. Nevertheless, the small subgroup of KIT- and DOG1.1-negative GISTs remains a diagnostic challenge, and mutational analysis may be helpful in this setting. However, because this subgroup is enriched for wild-type tumors (lacking mutations in either *KIT* or *PDGFRA*), one must often rely on traditional pathologic assessment in such cases.

Recently, Price and colleagues[66,67] proposed an apparently highly accurate two-gene classifier to differentiate GISTs from leiomyosarcomas, as well as to identify KIT-negative GISTs and those with weak or heterogeneous KIT expression. The proposed PCR-based assay depends on the identification of a gene set (*OBSCN* and *C9orf65*) identified through top-scoring pair analysis (a method able to identify a gene pair whose relative expression is reversed between two cancer types). The estimated accuracy of this test was approximately 98%.[66] Although this test appears promising, these findings have not yet been validated by independent groups or in a set of diagnostically problematic tumors equivocal by other standard criteria.

RISK ASSESSMENT IN GASTROINTESTINAL STROMAL TUMORS

Morphologic risk assessment in GISTs provides the basis for clinical management and optimal patient care. The vast majority of studies of GISTs suggest that the two most important prognostic features to assess the risk of aggressive behavior in a primary GIST are mitotic activity and tumor size. These two features were the foundation of the consensus approach for risk assessment in GISTs published by Fletcher and colleagues[1,68] in 2002 (**Table 1**). Subsequent data collected by Miettinen and colleagues,[22,39,40,69] analyzing large series of GISTs, confirmed that tumor size and mitotic activity are essential prognostic parameters; they proposed additional new parameters in the evaluation of the clinical behavior of GISTs. According to the new guidelines,[12] GISTs smaller than 2 cm without significant mitotic activity (ie, <5 per 50 high-power fields) can be regarded as essentially benign. However, in the

Table 1 Proposed approach for defining risk of aggressive behavior in GISTs		
Risk Level	**Size[a]**	**Mitotic Count[b]**
Very low risk	<2 cm	<5/50 HPF
Low risk	2–5 cm	<5/50 HPF
Intermediate risk	<5 cm	6–10/50 HPF
	5–10 cm	<5/50 HPF
High risk	>5 cm	>5/50 HPF
	>10 cm	Any mitotic rate
	Any size	>10/50HPF

[a] Size represents the single largest dimension. Admittedly, this may vary somewhat between before fixation and after fixation and between observers. There is a general but poorly defined sense that perhaps the size threshold for aggressive behavior should be 1 cm to 2 cm less in the small bowel than elsewhere.

[b] Ideally, mitotic count should be standardized according to surface area examined (based on size of high-power fields), but there are no agreed-on definitions in this regard. Despite inevitable subjectivity in recognition of mitoses and variability in the area of high power fields, such mitotic counts still prove useful.

Adapted from Fletcher CD, Berman JJ, Corless C, et al. Diagnosis of gastrointestinal stromal tumors: A consensus approach. Hum Pathol 2002;33(5):464; with permission.

2002 consensus guidelines,[1] all GISTs were proposed to have some, albeit miniscule in some cases, malignant potential. Therefore, these small GISTs should be considered as a gray zone and more work is needed with regard to this specific group. These differences in opinion may boil down to one of preference or perception—is a tumor benign because it almost never metastasizes or malignant because it can very rarely metastasize? Obviously, the risk for GIST would be best defined as a continuous variable, but the defined categories are clinically useful, even if artificially imposed. The next strongest parameter in these studies was tumor location. Miettinen and colleagues showed that small intestinal and rectal GISTs were more aggressive than gastric GISTs of similar size.[22,40,70,71] Therefore, mitotic activity, tumor size, and anatomic site are now the three proposed parameters for risk assessment in GISTs according to the 2007 National Comprehensive Cancer Network (NCCN) guidelines (**Table 2**).[12]

Additional Proposed Pathologic Prognostic Parameters

Additional morphology-based prognostic parameters not included in the NCCN guidelines have been proposed by Miettinen and colleagues. Although these parameters are not universally used or accepted, their findings are certainly of interest and are discussed below.

Gastric Gastrointestinal Stromal Tumors

Miettinen and colleagues[22] investigated 1765 gastric GISTs from the pre-imatinib era and proposed that GISTs showing spindle cell morphology have a worse prognosis than epithelioid GISTs at this anatomic site. They also proposed that evaluating the grade [mild, moderate, or high (sarcomatous)] and distribution (focal or diffuse) of nuclear atypia could aid in prognostication. Although it seems plausible that diffuse high-grade atypia would be associated with a worse prognosis, the grading of atypia is subjective, and its reproducibility among pathologists remains questionable. Furthermore, high-grade nuclear atypia is associated with a higher mitotic index in

Table 2
Risk stratification of primary GIST by mitotic index, size and site

Tumor Parameters		Risk of Progressive Disease(%)[a]			
	Size	Gastric	Duodenum	Jejunum/Ileum	Rectum
Mitotic Index ≤5 per 50 hpf	≤2 cm	None	None	None	None
	>2 ≤5 cm	Very low (1.9)	Low (8.3)	Low (4.3)	Low (8.5)
	>5 ≤10 cm	Low (3.6)	(Insuff. data)	Moderate (24)	(Insuff. data)
	>10 cm	Moderate (10)	High (34)	High (52)	High (57)
Mitotic Index >5 per 50 hpf	≤2 cm	None[b]	(Insuff. data)	High[b]	High (54)
	>2 ≤5 cm	Moderate (16)	High (50)	High (73)	High (52)
	>5 ≤10 cm	High (55)	(Insuff. data)	High (85)	(Insuff. data)
	>10 cm	High (86)	High (86)	High (90)	High (71)

Data based on long-term follow-up of 1055 gastric, 629 small intestinal, 144 duodenal and 111 rectal GISTs.[22,40]

Abbreviation: Insuff. data, insufficient data available to characterize.
[a] Defined as metastasis or tumor-related death.
[b] Denotes small numbers of cases.

Adapted from Miettinen M, Lasota J. Gastrointestinal stromal tumors: pathology and prognosis at different sites. Semin Diagn Pathol 2006;23(2):70–83; with permission.

most cases. The independent significance of nuclear grade should be evaluated in further studies. Other parameters associated with a worse prognosis are coagulative necrosis, ulceration, and mucosal invasion, features that are easily reproducible. Similarly, whether these parameters add additional prognostic information beyond the NCCN guidelines remains uncertain and requires further study with multivariate analysis. A parameter proposed to be associated with a favorable prognosis was nuclear palisading, though this feature is relatively infrequently encountered. Muscle invasion, liquefactive necrosis, or other growth patterns were not associated with clinical behavior in GISTs located in the stomach.

Small Intestinal Gastrointestinal Stromal Tumors

According to the largest study of GISTs occurring in the small intestine, including 906 cases, 86% of small intestinal GISTs show spindle cell morphology, 5% epithelioid morphology, and 9% mixed morphology.[40] Proposed parameters associated with significantly worse prognosis in univariate analysis were epithelioid and mixed cytomorphology, diffuse nuclear atypia, coagulative necrosis, ulceration, mucosal invasion, and an organoid paraganglioma-like nested growth pattern.[40] With the exception of diffuse nuclear atypia, which is a subjective parameter that may not be reproducible among pathologists, these parameters could be included in a pathology report to generate additional information for risk assessment. However, because some of these parameters were associated with higher mitotic activity, it remains unclear whether they provide additional prognostic information independent of size and mitotic index. Parameters associated with a favorable prognosis were skeinoid fibers and nuclear palisading.

PROPOSED PROGNOSTICALLY VALUABLE IMMUNOHISTOCHEMICAL MARKERS IN GASTROINTESTINAL STROMAL TUMORS

The tumor suppressor gene *CDKN2A* (p16) on chromosome 9p21 is an important cell cycle inhibitor that has been shown to be inactivated in a significant proportion of malignancies.[72–77] Immunohistochemistry has been used to assess p16 status, and the down-regulation of p16 correlates with aggressive behavior in GISTs, apparently even in tumors that are classified as low risk according to standard morphologic parameters.[73,74,76]

Another cell cycle inhibitor, p27, has been shown to be down-regulated in malignant GISTs, and up-regulation of cell cycle regulatory proteins (cyclins B1, D and E; cdc2, CDK2, CDK4 and CDK6), as well as increased expression of p53, RB, and cyclin A by immunohistochemistry, have been proposed to be more common in high-risk GISTs.[74,76,78–81]

The caveat to the use of these markers for routine clinical purposes is the fact that standardized protocols for interpretation of these markers have not yet been established. To date, p16 seems to be a promising independent marker for risk evaluation in GISTs. However, recently Steigen and colleagues[77] demonstrated that increased p16 expression, rather than down-regulation, was associated with an unfavorable prognosis. Additional studies are needed to clarify this relationship.

A recent publication indicates that vascular endothelial growth factor may be a negative prognostic indicator in GIST.[82] This factor seemed to be associated with poor response to imatinib in this study independent of *KIT* mutation type, and thus may be more of a biomarker for therapeutic response than a prognostic marker of the natural history of GIST. Further studies are needed to confirm this finding.

DIFFERENTIAL DIAGNOSIS

The main differential diagnostic considerations for spindle cell GISTs are smooth muscle tumors, desmoid fibromatosis, schwannoma, inflammatory myofibroblastic tumor, inflammatory fibroid polyp, solitary fibrous tumor, and synovial sarcoma (**Fig. 8**). Importantly, all of these tumor types are consistently negative for KIT. Mural leiomyomas occur most commonly in the esophagus, and at this location are more common than GISTs, with a 3-to-1 ratio.[83] In contrast to the syncytial appearance of spindle cell GISTs, smooth muscle tumors show more brightly eosinophilic cytoplasm and better defined cell borders. SMA and caldesmon are expressed in both GISTs and smooth muscle tumors, and are therefore of limited use in the differential diagnosis of these tumor types. In contrast, desmin is relatively specific for smooth muscle tumors and is rarely expressed in spindle-cell GISTs (see **Fig. 8A**). Gastrointestinal schwannomas often show a distinctive peripheral cuff of lymphocytes and strongly express S-100 protein in the vast majority of neoplastic cells (see **Fig. 8B**).[84] Furthermore, GISTs consistently lack the expression of glial fibrillary acidic protein, a marker commonly expressed in gastrointestinal schwannomas. Intra-abdominal desmoid fibromatosis is composed of long sweeping fascicles of spindle cells usually set within a collagenous matrix. Immunohistochemistry reveals nuclear β-catenin positivity in the vast majority of cases (see **Fig. 8C**).[85–87] Inflammatory myofibroblastic tumors mainly occur in children and young adults. They are cellular, fascicular fibroblastic/myofibroblastic tumors with a prominent inflammatory infiltrate composed chiefly of plasma cells (see **Fig. 8D**). Diffuse expression of SMA is common. ALK expression by immunohistochemistry can facilitate the diagnosis,[88] but is seen in

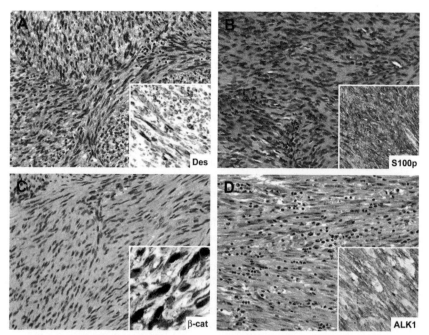

Fig. 8. Potential spindle cell GIST mimics. (*A*) Leiomyosarcoma (200×), desmin inset; (*B*) schwannoma (200×), S-100 protein inset; (*C*) desmoid fibromatosis (200×), nuclear β-catenin inset; (*D*) inflammatory myofibroblastic tumor (200×), ALK-1 inset.

only 50% of cases (mostly in children).[89] Inflammatory fibroid polyps usually present as ulcerated intraluminal polyps. These lesions are highly vascular, showing a myxoid granulation tissue-like stroma containing numerous eosinophils. Fibroblasts typically show an onion skin-like orientation around blood vessels and usually express CD34. Solitary fibrous tumors (SFTs) are characterized by their branching hemangiopericytoma-like vessels and a patternless architecture in combination with hypercellular and hypocellular areas. SFTs express CD34 and often CD99.[90] Synovial sarcoma is rarely encountered in the GI tract. In the monophasic form, patchy reactivity for cytokeratins and epilethial membrane antigen is helpful. Molecular demonstration of the t(X;18) (p11;q11) chromosomal translocation present in virtually all cases is diagnostic.[91]

The main differential diagnosis of epithelioid GISTs includes glomus tumors, neuroendocrine carcinoma, epithelioid leiomyosarcoma, metastatic melanoma, epithelioid malignant peripheral nerve sheath tumor (MPNST), and clear cell sarcoma. Glomus tumors rarely occur in the GI tract, where they are almost exclusively seen in the stomach. Morphologically and immunohistochemically, these tumors are identical to glomus tumors in other locations, strongly express SMA, but are negative for desmin, S-100 protein, and KIT. Neuroendocrine carcinomas are usually reactive for cytokeratins and also express neuroendocrine markers, such as synaptophysin and chromogranin. Epithelioid leiomyosarcomas express the smooth muscle markers SMA, desmin, and caldesmon, but do not express KIT. Desmin is only rarely expressed in GISTs, though KIT-negative gastric epithelioid GISTs can express desmin in approximately one-third of cases.[54] Therefore, in this setting, mutational testing should be considered to confirm the diagnosis. Metastatic melanoma and clear cell sarcoma express S-100 protein; the former also often expresses melanocytic markers. Primary gastrointestinal clear cell sarcomas often lack melanocytic differentiation, unlike their soft-tissue counterparts.[92] Although some metastatic melanomas express KIT,[48] the additional expression of melanocytic markers and clinical history will facilitate the correct diagnosis. Furthermore, EWSR1 (22q12) rearrangements with either CREB1 (2q32) or ATF1 (12q13) are seen in the majority of primary gastrointestinal clear cell sarcomas.[93,94] Epithelioid MPNSTs lack KIT expression but usually strongly express S-100 protein in the absence of second-line melanoma markers.

MOLECULAR CLASSIFICATION OF GASTROINTESTINAL STROMAL TUMORS

Objective clinical response to imatinib has been shown to depend on the type of RTK mutation, and a molecular classification of GISTs has been proposed.[95,96] Based on the results of clinical trials (phase I–III)[12] investigating over 700 genotyped GISTs,[11,97,98] the objective response rate for KIT exon 11 mutant GISTs is 72% to 86%, compared with 38% to 48% for KIT exon 9 mutations, and up to 28% for wild-type GISTs.[11,97–99] Primary resistance to imatinib has been likewise demonstrated in 5% of GISTs showing KIT exon 11 mutation and in 16% and 23% of KIT exon 9 mutant and KIT wild-type GISTs, respectively.[11,97,98] Similarly, the most common PDGFRA mutation (D842V) is completely resistant to imatinib.[11,55,100] Other PDGFRA mutations appear to show partial response to imatinib; however, given the rarity of these tumors, data are limited.

Standard therapy for patients with advanced metastatic GIST has been an oral dose of 400 mg imatinib per day, regardless of the underlying mutation. However, recent studies suggest that patients with tumors harboring a KIT exon 9 mutation derive greater benefit from treatment with higher doses of imatinib (800 mg per day).[11,12,97,98] Furthermore, very recent observations suggest that sunitinib could be a better first-line treatment option for patients with KIT exon 9 mutant or KIT wild-type GISTs,[101] and other novel TKIs are currently being evaluated.

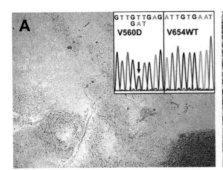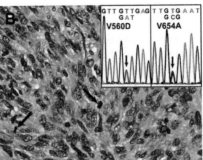

Fig. 9. Imatinib mesylate resistance mutations. (A) Treated GIST, inset exon 11 mutation and exon 13 wild-type; the lower right corner shows a resistant focus. (B) Higher power of resistant GIST focus with mitoses denoted by arrows (400×), showing retention of the initial exon 11 mutation and an acquired exon 13 (V654A) resistance mutation (inset).

Routine mutational testing of all GISTs is controversial, but becoming increasingly employed in large treatment centers. There is emerging consensus that mutational testing should be considered for unresectable and metastatic GISTs before treatment with imatinib and for high-risk primary tumors. Although most institutions are now treating patients with imatinib as first-line therapy, irrespective of the mutational status, this treatment regime will certainly change in the future as the TKI armamentarium increases and additional studies of efficacy stratified by genotype are completed. Mutational testing for secondary mutations associated with acquired resistance to imatinib is an area of active research and growing clinical importance, given the number of patients being chronically treated with this agent (**Fig. 9**). The authors recently demonstrated striking intra- and inter-lesional heterogeneity in TKI-resistance mechanisms.[102] With regard to treatment approches, application of combinations of additional and newer generation KIT and PDGFRA TKIs may provide efficacy in this setting, but additional investigation is needed in this regard. These subjects are further discussed elsewhere in this issue.

SUMMARY

There is a wide morphologic spectrum of GISTs, but virtually all cases are amenable to the proposed primary parameters for risk assessment (size, mitotic index, and anatomic site). In addition to the common morphologic subgroups of GIST (spindle cell, epithelioid, and mixed), unusual morphologic variants, morphologic changes after TKI treatment, and treatment effects on GISTs are encountered. Promising new immunohistochemical markers (such as DOG1.1) will likely be diagnostically valuable, especially in GISTs lacking KIT expression. Although the routine molecular classification of GISTs for clinical management is not universally accepted, there are certainly instances where this is valuable and there is utility for testing in cases where immunohistochemistry is insufficient to confirm the diagnosis.

ACKNOWLEDGMENTS

The authors thank Kim Vu for expert assistance in figure production and Lindsey P. Lyle for gross photography. The authors also thank Dr. Chris Corless of Oregon Health and Science University, Portland, Oregon for the adapted and corrected 2007 NCCN risk assessment chart.

REFERENCES

1. Fletcher CD, Berman JJ, Corless C, et al. Diagnosis of gastrointestinal stromal tumors: a consensus approach. Hum Pathol 2002;33(5):459–65.
2. Mazur MT, Clark HB. Gastric stromal tumors. Reappraisal of histogenesis. Am J Surg Pathol 1983;7(6):507–19.
3. Miettinen M, Virolainen M, Maarit Sarlomo R, et al. Gastrointestinal stromal tumors—value of CD34 antigen in their identification and separation from true leiomyomas and schwannomas. Am J Surg Pathol 1995;19(2):207–16.
4. Huizinga JD, Thuneberg L, Kluppel M, et al. W/kit gene required for interstitial cells of Cajal and for intestinal pacemaker activity. Nature 1995;373(6512): 347–9.
5. Hirota S, Isozaki K, Moriyama Y, et al. Gain-of-function mutations of c-kit in human gastrointestinal stromal tumors. Science 1998;279(5350):577–80.
6. Kindblom L, Ramotti H, Aldenborg F, et al. Gastrointestinal pacemaker cell tumor (GIPACT): gastrointestinal stromal tumors show phenotypic characteristics of the interstitial cells of Cajal. Am J Pathol 1998;152(5):259–69.
7. Robinson TL, Sircar K, Hewlett BR, et al. Gastrointestinal stromal tumors may originate from a subset of CD34-positive interstitial cells of Cajal. Am J Pathol 2000;156(4):1157–63.
8. Isozaki K, Hirota S, Nakama A, et al. Disturbed intestinal movement, bile reflux to the stomach, and deficiency of c-kit-expressing cells in Ws/Ws mutant rats. Gastroenterology 1995;109(2):456–64.
9. Der-Silaphet T, Malysz J, Hagel S, et al. Interstitial cells of Cajal direct normal propulsive contractile activity in the mouse small intestine. Gastroenterology 1998;114(4):724–36.
10. Heinrich MC, Corless CL, Duensing A, et al. PDGFRA activating mutations in gastrointestinal stromal tumors. Science 2003;299(5607):708–10.
11. Heinrich MC, Corless CL, Demetri GD, et al. Kinase mutations and imatinib response in patients with metastatic gastrointestinal stromal tumor. J Clin Oncol 2003;21(23):4342–9.
12. Demetri GD, Benjamin RS, Blanke CD, et al. NCCN Task Force report: management of patients with gastrointestinal stromal tumor (GIST)–update of the NCCN clinical practice guidelines. J Natl Compr Canc Netw 2007;5(Suppl 2):S1–29 [quiz S30].
13. Edmonson JH, Marks RS, Buckner JC, et al. Contrast of response to dacarbazine, mitomycin, doxorubicin, and cisplatin (DMAP) plus GM-CSF between patients with advanced malignant gastrointestinal stromal tumors and patients with other advanced leiomyosarcomas. Cancer Invest 2002;20(5–6):605–12.
14. Goettsch WG, Bos SD, Breekveldt-Postma N, et al. Incidence of gastrointestinal stromal tumours is underestimated: results of a nation-wide study. Eur J Cancer 2005;41(18):2868–72.
15. Nilsson B, Bumming P, Meis-Kindblom JM, et al. Gastrointestinal stromal tumors: the incidence, prevalence, clinical course, and prognostication in the preimatinib mesylate era—a population-based study in western Sweden. Cancer 2005;103(4):821–9.
16. Tryggvason G, Gislason HG, Magnusson MK, et al. Gastrointestinal stromal tumors in Iceland, 1990–2003: the Icelandic GIST study, a population-based incidence and pathologic risk stratification study. Int J Cancer 2005;117(2):289–93.
17. Agaimy A, Wunsch PH, Hofstaedter F, et al. Minute gastric sclerosing stromal tumors (GIST tumorlets) are common in adults and frequently show c-KIT mutations. Am J Surg Pathol 2007;31(1):113–20.

18. Kawanowa K, Sakuma Y, Sakurai S, et al. High incidence of microscopic gastrointestinal stromal tumors in the stomach. Hum Pathol 2006;37(12):1527–35.

19. Abraham SC, Krasinskas AM, Hofstetter WL, et al. "Seedling" mesenchymal tumors (gastrointestinal stromal tumors and leiomyomas) are common incidental tumors of the esophagogastric junction. Am J Surg Pathol 2007;31(11):1629–35.

20. Agaimy A, Wunsch PH, Dirnhofer S, et al. Microscopic gastrointestinal stromal tumors in esophageal and intestinal surgical resection specimens: a clinicopathologic, immunohistochemical, and molecular study of 19 lesions. Am J Surg Pathol 2008;32(6):867–73.

21. Corless CL, McGreevey L, Haley A, et al. KIT mutations are common in incidental gastrointestinal stromal tumors one centimeter or less in size. Am J Pathol 2002;160(5):1567–72.

22. Miettinen M, Sobin LH, Lasota J, et al. Gastrointestinal stromal tumors of the stomach: a clinicopathologic, immunohistochemical, and molecular genetic study of 1765 cases with long-term follow-up. Am J Surg Pathol 2005;29(1):52–68.

23. Prakash S, Sarran L, Socci N, et al. Gastrointestinal stromal tumors in children and young adults: a clinicopathologic, molecular, and genomic study of 15 cases and review of the literature. J Pediatr Hematol Oncol 2005;27(4):179–87.

24. Janeway KA, Liegl B, Harlow A, et al. Pediatric KIT wild-type and platelet-derived growth factor receptor alpha- wild-type gastrointestinal stromal tumors share KIT activation but not mechanisms of genetic progression with adult gastrointestinal stromal tumors. Cancer Res 2007;67(19):9084–8.

25. Beghini A, Tibiletti MG, Roversi G, et al. Germline mutation in the juxtamembrane domain of the kit gene in a family with gastrointestinal stromal tumors and urticaria pigmentosa. Cancer 2001;92(3):657–62.

26. Isozaki K, Terris B, Belghiti J, et al. Germline-activating mutation in the kinase domain of KIT gene in familial gastrointestinal stromal tumors. Am J Pathol 2000;157(5):1581–5.

27. Kang DY, Park CK, Choi JS, et al. Multiple gastrointestinal stromal tumors: Clinicopathologic and genetic analysis of 12 patients. Am J Surg Pathol 2007; 31(2):224–32.

28. Maeyama H, Hidaka E, Ota H, et al. Familial gastrointestinal stromal tumor with hyperpigmentation: association with a germline mutation of the c-kit gene. Gastroenterology 2001;120(1):210–5.

29. Nishida T, Hirota S, Taniguchi M, et al. Familial gastrointestinal stromal tumours with germline mutation of the KIT gene. Nat Genet 1998;19(4):323–4.

30. O'Riain C, Corless CL, Heinrich MC, et al. Gastrointestinal stromal tumors: insights from a new familial GIST kindred with unusual genetic and pathologic features. Am J Surg Pathol 2005;29(12):1680–3.

31. Kleinbaum EP, Lazar AJ, Tamborini E, et al. Clinical, histopathologic, molecular and therapeutic findings in a large kindred with gastrointestinal stromal tumor. Int J Cancer 2008;122(3):711–8.

32. Andersson J, Sihto H, Meis-Kindblom JM, et al. NF1-associated gastrointestinal stromal tumors have unique clinical, phenotypic, and genotypic characteristics. Am J Surg Pathol 2005;29(9):1170–6.

33. Maertens O, Prenen H, Debiec-Rychter M, et al. Molecular pathogenesis of multiple gastrointestinal stromal tumors in NF1 patients. Hum Mol Genet 2006; 15(6):1015–23.

34. Miettinen M, Fetsch JF, Sobin LH, et al. Gastrointestinal stromal tumors in patients with neurofibromatosis 1: a clinicopathologic and molecular genetic study of 45 cases. Am J Surg Pathol 2006;30(1):90–6.

35. Carney JA. Gastric stromal sarcoma, pulmonary chondroma, and extra-adrenal paraganglioma (Carney Triad). Natural history, adrenocortical component, and possible familial occurrence. Mayo Clin Proc 1999;74(6):543–52.

36. Carney JA, Stratakis CA. Familial paraganglioma and gastric stromal sarcoma: a new syndrome distinct from the Carney triad. Am J Med Genet 2002;108(2):132–9.

37. Pasini B, McWhinney SR, Bei T, et al. Clinical and molecular genetics of patients with the Carney-Stratakis syndrome and germline mutations of the genes coding for the succinate dehydrogenase subunits SDHB, SDHC, and SDHD. Eur J Hum Genet 2008;16(1):79–88.

38. DeMatteo RP, Lewis JJ, Leung D, et al. Two hundred gastrointestinal stromal tumors: recurrence patterns and prognostic factors for survival. Ann Surg 2000;231(1):51–8.

39. Miettinen M, Lasota J, Sobin LH, et al. Gastrointestinal stromal tumors of the stomach in children and young adults: a clinicopathologic, immunohistochemical, and molecular genetic study of 44 cases with long-term follow-up and review of the literature. Am J Surg Pathol 2005;29(10):1373–81.

40. Miettinen M, Makhlouf H, Sobin LH, et al. Gastrointestinal stromal tumors of the jejunum and ileum: a clinicopathologic, immunohistochemical, and molecular genetic study of 906 cases before imatinib with long-term follow-up. Am J Surg Pathol 2006;30(4):477–89.

41. Miettinen M, Monihan JM, Sarlomo-Rikala M, et al. Gastrointestinal stromal tumors/smooth muscle tumors (GISTs) primary in the omentum and mesentery: clinicopathologic and immunohistochemical study of 26 cases. Am J Surg Pathol 1999;23(9):1109–18.

42. Reith JD, Goldblum JR, Lyles RH, et al. Extragastrointestinal (soft tissue) stromal tumors: an analysis of 48 cases with emphasis on histologic predictors of outcome. Mod Pathol 2000;13(5):577–85.

43. Verma P, Corless C, Medeiros F, et al. Pleomorphic gastrointestinal stromal tumors: diagnostic and therapeutic implications. Mod Pathol 2005;18(Suppl 1):121A.

44. Antonescu CR, Hornick JL, Nielsen GP, et al. Dedifferentiation in gastrointestinal stromal tumor (GIST) to an anaplastic KIT-negative phenotype—a diagnostic pitfall. Mod Pathol 2007;20(Suppl 2):11A.

45. Pauwels P, Debiec-Rychter M, Stul M, et al. Changing phenotype of gastrointestinal stromal tumours under imatinib mesylate treatment: a potential diagnostic pitfall. Histopathology 2005;47(1):41–7.

46. Liegl B, Hornick JL, Antonescu C, et al. Rhabdomyosarcomatous differentiation in gastrointestinal stromal tumors after tyrosine kinase inhibitor therapy: a novel form of tumor progression. Am J Surg Pathol, in press [Epub ahead of print].

47. de Raedt T, Cools J, Debiec-Rychter M, et al. Intestinal neurofibromatosis is a subtype of familial GIST and results from a dominant activating mutation in PDGFRA. Gastroenterology 2006;131(6):1907–12.

48. Hornick JL, Fletcher CD. Immunohistochemical staining for KIT (CD117) in soft tissue sarcomas is very limited in distribution. Am J Clin Pathol 2002;117(2):188–93.

49. Hornick JL, Fletcher CD. The significance of KIT (CD117) in gastrointestinal stromal tumors. Int J Surg Pathol 2004;12(2):93–7.

50. Sarlomo-Rikala M, Kovatich A, Barusevicius A, et al. CD117: a sensitive marker for gastrointestinal stromal tumors that is more specific than CD34. Mod Pathol 1998;(11):728–34.

51. Debiec-Rychter M, Wasag B, Stul M, et al. Gastrointestinal stromal tumours (GISTs) negative for KIT (CD117 antigen) immunoreactivity. J Pathol 2004; 202(4):430–8.

52. Medeiros F, Corless CL, Duensing A, et al. KIT-negative gastrointestinal stromal tumors: proof of concept and therapeutic implications. Am J Surg Pathol 2004; 28(7):889–94.

53. Orosz Z, Tornoczky T, Sapi Z, et al. Gastrointestinal stromal tumors: a clinicopathologic and immunohistochemical study of 136 cases. Pathol Oncol Res 2005; 11(1):11–21.

54. Liegl B, Hornick JL, Corless C, et al. Monoclonal antibody DOG 1.1 shows higher sensitivity than KIT in the diagnosis of gastrointestinal stromal tumors, including unusual subtypes. Am J Surg Pathol, in press [Epub ahead of print].

55. Corless CL, Schroeder A, Griffith D, et al. PDGFRA mutations in gastrointestinal stromal tumors: frequency, spectrum and in vitro sensitivity to imatinib. J Clin Oncol 2005;23(23):5357–64.

56. Weisberg E, Wright RD, Jiang J, et al. Effects of PKC412, nilotinib, and imatinib against GIST-associated PDGFRA mutants with differential imatinib sensitivity. Gastroenterology 2006;131(6):1734–42.

57. Espinosa I, Lee CH, Kim MK, et al. A novel monoclonal antibody against DOG1 is a sensitive and specific marker for gastrointestinal stromal tumors. Am J Surg Pathol 2008;32(2):210–8.

58. West RB, Corless CL, Chen X, et al. The novel marker, DOG1, is expressed ubiquitously in gastrointestinal stromal tumors irrespective of KIT or PDGFRA mutation status. Am J Pathol 2004;165(1):107–13.

59. Blay P, Astudillo A, Buesa JM, et al. Protein kinase C theta is highly expressed in gastrointestinal stromal tumors but not in other mesenchymal neoplasias. Clin Cancer Res 2004;10(12 Pt 1):4089–95.

60. Duensing A, Joseph NE, Medeiros F, et al. Protein Kinase C theta (PKCtheta) expression and constitutive activation in gastrointestinal stromal tumors (GISTs). Cancer Res 2004;64(15):5127–31.

61. Lee HE, Kim MA, Lee HS, et al. Characteristics of KIT-negative gastrointestinal stromal tumors and diagnostic utility of protein kinase C theta immunostaining. J Clin Pathol 2008;61(6):722–9.

62. Rossi G, Valli R, Bertolini F, et al. PDGFR expression in differential diagnosis between KIT-negative gastrointestinal stromal tumours and other primary soft-tissue tumours of the gastrointestinal tract. Histopathology 2005;46(5):522–31.

63. Peterson MR, Piao Z, Weidner N, et al. Strong PDGFRA positivity is seen in GISTs but not in other intra-abdominal mesenchymal tumors: Immunohistochemical and mutational analyses. Appl Immunohistochem Mol Morphol 2006;14(4):390–6.

64. Zheng S, Chen LR, Wang HJ, et al. Analysis of mutation and expression of c-kit and PDGFR-alpha gene in gastrointestinal stromal tumor. Hepatogastroenterology 2007;54(80):2285–90.

65. Miselli F, Millefanti C, Conca E, et al. PDGFRA immunostaining can help in the diagnosis of gastrointestinal stromal tumors. Am J Surg Pathol 2008;32(5):738–43.

66. Price ND, Trent J, El-Naggar AK, et al. Highly accurate two-gene classifier for differentiating gastrointestinal stromal tumors and leiomyosarcomas. Proc Natl Acad Sci U S A 2007;104(9):3414–9.

67. Trent JC, Lazar AJ, Zhang W, et al. Molecular approaches to resolve diagnostic dilemmas: the case of gastrointestinal stromal tumor and leiomyosarcoma. Future Oncol 2007;3(6):629–37.

68. Fletcher CD, Berman JJ, Corless C, et al. Diagnosis of gastrointestinal stromal tumors: a consensus approach. Int J Surg Pathol 2002;10(2):81–9.

69. Miettinen M, Lasota J. Gastrointestinal stromal tumors: pathology and prognosis at different sites. Semin Diagn Pathol 2006;23(2):70–83.

70. Miettinen M, Kopczynski J, Makhlouf HR, et al. Gastrointestinal stromal tumors, intramural leiomyomas, and leiomyosarcomas in the duodenum: a clinicopathologic, immunohistochemical, and molecular genetic study of 167 cases. Am J Surg Pathol 2003;27(5):625–41.

71. Miettinen M, Lasota J. Gastrointestinal stromal tumors: review on morphology, molecular pathology, prognosis, and differential diagnosis. Arch Pathol Lab Med 2006;130(10):1466–78.

72. Perrone F, Tamborini E, Dagrada GP, et al. 9p21 locus analysis in high-risk gastrointestinal stromal tumors characterized for c-kit and platelet-derived growth factor receptor alpha gene alterations. Cancer 2005;104(1):159–69.

73. Ricci R, Arena V, Castri F, et al. Role of p16/INK4a in gastrointestinal stromal tumor progression. Am J Clin Pathol 2004;122(1):35–43.

74. Sabah M, Cummins R, Leader M, et al. Loss of heterozygosity of chromosome 9p and loss of p16INK4A expression are associated with malignant gastrointestinal stromal tumors. Mod Pathol 2004;17(11):1364–71.

75. Schneider-Stock R, Boltze C, Lasota J, et al. High prognostic value of p16INK4 alterations in gastrointestinal stromal tumors. J Clin Oncol 2003;21(9):1688–97.

76. Schneider-Stock R, Boltze C, Lasota J, et al. Loss of p16 protein defines high-risk patients with gastrointestinal stromal tumors: a tissue microarray study. Clin Cancer Res 2005;11(2 Pt 1):638–45.

77. Steigen SE, Bjerkehagen B, Haugland HK, et al. Diagnostic and prognostic markers for gastrointestinal stromal tumors in Norway. Mod Pathol 2008;21(1): 46–53.

78. Feakins RM. The expression of p53 and bcl-2 in gastrointestinal stromal tumours is associated with anatomical site, and p53 expression is associated with grade and clinical outcome. Histopathology 2005;46(3):270–9.

79. Nemoto Y, Mikami T, Hana K, et al. Correlation of enhanced cell turnover with prognosis of gastrointestinal stromal tumors of the stomach: relevance of cellularity and p27kip1. Pathol Int 2006;56(12):724–31.

80. Pruneri G, Mazzarol G, Fabris S, et al. Cyclin D3 immunoreactivity in gastrointestinal stromal tumors is independent of cyclin D3 gene amplification and is associated with nuclear p27 accumulation. Mod Pathol 2003;16(9):886–92.

81. Tornillo L, Duchini G, Carafa V, et al. Patterns of gene amplification in gastrointestinal stromal tumors (GIST). Lab Invest 2005;85(7):921–31.

82. McAuliffe JC, Lazar AJ, Yang D, et al. Association of intratumoral vascular endothelial growth factor expression and clinical outcome for patients with gastrointestinal stromal tumors treated with imatinib mesylate. Clin Cancer Res 2007; 13(22 Pt 1):6727–34.

83. Miettinen M, Sarlomo-Rikala M, Sobin LH, et al. Esophageal stromal tumors: a clinicopathologic, immunohistochemical, and molecular genetic study of 17 cases and comparison with esophageal leiomyomas and leiomyosarcomas. Am J Surg Pathol 2000;24(2):211–22.

84. Sarlomo-Rikala M, Miettinen M. Gastric schwannoma—a clinicopathological analysis of six cases. Histopathology 1995;27(4):355–60.

85. Carlson JW, Fletcher CD. Immunohistochemistry for beta-catenin in the differential diagnosis of spindle cell lesions: analysis of a series and review of the literature. Histopathology 2007;51(4):509–14.

86. Montgomery E, Torbenson MS, Kaushal M, et al. Beta-catenin immunohistochemistry separates mesenteric fibromatosis from gastrointestinal stromal tumor and sclerosing mesenteritis. Am J Surg Pathol 2002;26(10):1296–301.

87. Lazar AJ, Tuvin D, Hajibashi S, et al. Specific mutations in the beta-catenin gene (CTNNB1) correlate with local recurrence in sporadic desmoid tumors. Am J Pathol 2008;173(5):1518–27.

88. Cessna MH, Zhou H, Sanger WG, et al. Expression of ALK1 and p80 in inflammatory myofibroblastic tumor and its mesenchymal mimics: a study of 135 cases. Mod Pathol 2002;15(9):931–8.

89. Gleason BC, Hornick JL. Inflammatory myofibroblastic tumours: where are we now? J Clin Pathol Apr 2008;61(4):428–37.

90. WHO. Pathology and genetics tumors of soft tissue and bone. Lyon: IARCPress; 2002.

91. Lazar A, Abruzzo LV, Pollock RE, et al. Molecular diagnosis of sarcomas: chromosomal translocations in sarcomas. Arch Pathol Lab Med 2006;130(8): 1199–207.

92. Agaram NP, Baren A, Arkun K, et al. Comparative ultrastructural analysis and KIT/PDGFRA genotype in 125 gastrointestinal stromal tumors. Ultrastruct Pathol 2006;30(6):443–52.

93. Antonescu CR, Nafa K, Segal NH, et al. EWS-CREB1: a recurrent variant fusion in clear cell sarcoma—association with gastrointestinal location and absence of melanocytic differentiation. Clin Cancer Res 2006;12(18):5356–62.

94. Lyle PL, Amato CM, Fitzpatrick JE, et al. Gastrointestinal melanoma or clear cell sarcoma? Molecular evaluation of 7 cases previously diagnosed as malignant melanoma. Am J Surg Pathol 2008;32(6):858–66.

95. Corless CL, Fletcher JA, Heinrich MC, et al. Biology of gastrointestinal stromal tumors. J Clin Oncol 2004;22(18):3813–25.

96. Corless CL, Heinrich MC. Molecular pathobiology of gastrointestinal stromal sarcomas. Annu Rev Pathol 2008;3:557–86.

97. Debiec-Rychter M, Sciot R, Le Cesne A, et al. KIT mutations and dose selection for imatinib in patients with advanced gastrointestinal stromal tumours. Eur J Cancer 2006;42(8):1093–103.

98. Heinrich MC, Corless CL, Blanke CD, et al. Molecular correlates of imatinib resistance in gastrointestinal stromal tumors. J Clin Oncol 2006;24(29):4764–74.

99. Blanke CD, Demetri GD, von Mehren M, et al. Long-term results from a randomized phase II trial of standard- versus higher-dose imatinib mesylate for patients with unresectable or metastatic gastrointestinal stromal tumors expressing KIT. J Clin Oncol 2008;26(4):620–5.

100. Hirota S, Ohashi A, Nishida T, et al. Gain-of-function mutations of platelet-derived growth factor receptor alpha gene in gastrointestinal stromal tumors. Gastroenterology 2003;125(3):660–7.

101. Li FP, Fletcher JA, Heinrich MC, et al. Familial gastrointestinal stromal tumor syndrome: phenotypic and molecular features in a kindred. J Clin Oncol 2005;23(12):2735–43.

102. Liegl B, Kepten I, Le C, et al. Heterogeneity of kinase inhibitor resistance mechanisms in GIST. J Pathol 2008;216(1):64–74.

Gastrointestinal Stromal Tumor: A Clinical Overview

Richard Quek, MD[a,b], Suzanne George, MD[a,c],*

KEYWORDS

- Gastrointestinal stromal tumors • GIST • Review
- Imatinib • Sunitinib • Tyrosine kinase inhibitor

HISTORICAL PERSPECTIVE

Following descriptions in the 1940s by Stout and others, stromal tumors arising from the gastrointestinal tract were classified as smooth muscle neoplasms.[1,2] These rare tumors were classified as various entities including leiomyosarcoma, leiomyoblastoma and bizarre leiomyoma, until, at least, the 1960s. With the advent of electron microscopy (EM) in the late 1960s, smooth muscle features were seen only in occasional GIST cells, raising into question the smooth muscle origin of this entity.[3,4] In addition, several authors reported ultrastructural features reminiscent of autonomic nerve structures, with schwannian and neuroaxonal characteristics, in tumor specimens microscopically indistinguishable from GIST.[5]

With the introduction of immunohistochemistry in the early 1980s, it was soon appreciated that many of these tumors lacked immunophenotypic features of smooth muscle, and conversely, a proportion of tumors stained positively for S-100 protein, a marker for neuroectodermal differentiation.[6] This led Mazur and Clark to suggest the myenteric nervous system as a possible cell of origin and to introduce a more generic term, "stromal tumor." In 1989, a distinctive subset of gastrointestinal tumors showing autonomic neural features was described and termed "plexosarcoma"[7] and subsequently became better known as gastrointestinal autonomic nerve tumor (GANT).[8] By the early 1990s, there was considerable confusion as to the lines of

Dr Suzanne George has served on advisory boards for and received research funding from Pfizer.

[a] Center for Sarcoma and Bone Oncology, Dana-Farber Cancer Institute, 44 Binney Street, Boston, MA 02115, USA

[b] Department of Medical Oncology, National Cancer Centre Singapore, 11 Hospital Drive, Singapore 169610, Singapore

[c] Harvard Medical School, Boston, MA, USA

* Corresponding author. Center for Sarcoma and Bone Oncology, Dana-Farber Cancer Institute, 44 Binney Street, Boston, MA 02115.

E-mail address: sgeorge2@partners.org (S. George).

Hematol Oncol Clin N Am 23 (2009) 69–78

doi:10.1016/j.hoc.2008.11.006

0889-8588/08/$ – see front matter © 2009 Elsevier Inc. All rights reserved.

differentiation of these tumors. Some were obviously neurogenic, some myogenic, others displayed bidirectional differentiation and a subgroup with null phenotype. To further complicate matters, there was a distinct lack of histologic prognostication methods, with great difficulty classifying GISTs even into benign and malignant categories. Tumors showing the usual histologic criteria for malignancy did not uniformly behave aggressively, and on the other hand, some tumors with benign features gave rise to metastases.

From 1994, it became apparent that a significant proportion of GANTs were immunopositive for CD34, and for a while, CD34 was hailed as the marker for GIST.[9,10] This finding also raised the possibility that GIST might be related to the interstitial cells of Cajal (ICC) on the basis of CD34 immunopositivity. Interstitial cells of Cajal, sometimes known as the pacemaker cells of the gastrointestinal tract, form the interface between the autonomic nervous system and the smooth muscle. They possess the immunophenotypic and ultrastructural characteristics of both the neural and smooth muscle elements. However, over the next several years, it also became apparent that not more than 70% of GIST cases were truly positive for CD34. This was further confounded by the fact that Schwann cell, and other smooth muscle tumors, were also variably CD34 positive, thus obviating the diagnostic efficacy of CD34. Up until 1998, it was unclear what the cell of origin GIST derived from, how best to accurately diagnose GIST, or even to distinguish malignant from benign GIST. In parallel to developments in GIST, by the mid-1990s, various reports emerged describing gain-of-function mutations, and consequently, constitutive activation of KIT receptors in several human tumor mast cell lines.[11,12]

Finally in 1998, in a landmark publication, Hirota and colleagues[13] made two key discoveries: a near-universal expression of KIT in GIST and the presence of activating c-Kit mutations in GISTs. In Hirota's series of 49 GIST samples, 94% of cases expressed KIT. Mutations in the juxtamembrane domain of c-KIT were detected in five of six samples of GISTs, resulting in constitutive ligand-independent activation of the KIT receptor tyrosine kinase. The oncogenic role of KIT was confirmed when stable transfection of the mutant c-KIT cDNAs induced malignant transformation of murine lymphoid cells. In addition, 82% (40 of 49) of GISTs were CD34-positive and 78% (38 of 49) were positive for both CD34 and KIT. ICC were also found to be positive for both KIT and CD34, suggesting close morphologic relations between ICC and GIST. In the same year, work by Kindblom and colleagues[14] corroborated findings from Hirota and colleagues, showing that 78 of 78 GISTs studied were immunoreactive for KIT, and shared striking ultrastructural and immunophenotypic similarities with ICC. This work again supported the hypothesis that GIST may indeed develop from stem cells that differentiate toward ICC phenotype and confirmed KIT as an accurate diagnostic tool for GIST.

The next decade saw phenomenal growth in the understanding of GIST biology and therapeutics, beginning with a single patient with multiply treated, advanced refractory GIST, displaying early, rapid, and sustained response to a small molecule tyrosine kinase inhibitor (TKI) with potent activity against the transmembrane receptor KIT, ABL kinase and chimeric BCR-ABL fusion oncoprotein product of chronic myeloid leukemia, imatinib.[15] Imatinib occupies the ATP binding pocket of KIT, thereby preventing substrate phosphorylation, downstream signaling, and thereby inhibiting cell proliferation and survival. The remarkable, early clinical results led to the conduct of large-scale, rationally designed clinical trials of imatinib in patients with metastatic or unresectable GIST, aided by accurate diagnoses using CD117 expression (a marker of KIT-receptor tyrosine kinase), ultimately confirming the benefit and subsequent approval of imatinib in this indication by the US Food and Drug Administration in

February 2002.[16] Median progression-free survival of GIST patients on first-line imatinib is between 18- to -24 months. At the time of imatinib failure, sunitinib has
successfully demonstrated clinical activity in an international randomized placebo-
controlled phase 3 trial, leading to its approval in January 26, 2006, for use in patients
with imatinib-refractory or intolerant GIST.[17]

EPIDEMIOLOGY

Gastrointestinal stromal tumors represents about 5% of all sarcomas[18] and is the
most common (80%) mesenchymal neoplasm of the gastrointestinal tract.[19] Using
a Swedish population-based study, the annual incidence of GIST is estimated to be
14.5 per million and prevalence 129 per million,[20] with as many as 5000 to 6000
new cases per year in the United States.[21] Median age of onset is about 60 with no
gender predilection. GISTs may occasionally affect children and rare familial cases
have been reported in the literature, but the vast majority of cases are sporadic in
nature and risk factors are relatively unknown.

CLINICAL FEATURES

From a large population-based study, about one third of GIST cases were detected
incidentally, with approximately 20% found during surgery for other unrelated condition and remaining 10% found at autopsy.[20] The majority of GISTs, 50% to 60%, arise
in the stomach, 20% to 30% in the small bowel, 10% in the large bowel, 5% in the
esophagus and 5% from elsewhere in the abdominal cavity (eg, mesentery,
omentum).[21] A peculiar feature of GIST is that it is an essentially intra-abdominal
disease for the length of its natural history. Fifteen to 47% of patients present with
overt metastatic disease.[18,22] Common sites of metastases include liver, peritoneum
and omentum. Unlike adenocarcinoma, lymph node metastases are rare. In contrast
to other sarcomas, lung and bone metastases are unusual and appear late in the
course of disease, if at all. Brain metastases are exceedingly rare. For symptomatic
cases, presenting symptoms are invariably related to the gastrointestinal tract or
mass effect within the abdominal cavity, and include vague abdominal discomfort,
early satiety, palpable abdominal mass, or secondary symptoms of tumor bleeding
and associated anemia, bowel obstruction or perforation and dysphagia. Ensuing
investigations include appropriate radiological imaging with either computed tomography (CT) or magnetic resonance imaging (MRI) scans of the abdominopelvic cavity,
or functional imaging with positron emission tomography (PET), and endoscopies as
indicated.

RISK STRATIFICATION

For many years, there was little consensus on how best to distinguish benign from
malignant GIST. As alluded to earlier in this discussion, some tumors with morphologically malignant features did not display the expected aggressive behavior and some
tumors with histologically benign features develop metastases, sometimes years later.
Most experts now consider all GISTs to have malignant potential, instead of segre-
gating them into distinct categories of benign and malignant. Many factors have
been extensively studied and proposed to predict for outcome, but tumor size and
mitotic rate are the two most widely accepted indices, stratifying patients into four
risk groups.[21] Anatomic location of primary GIST tumor is also recognized as an independent prognostic factor,[23] with small bowel lesions carrying a higher risk of progression than gastric primaries of similar size and mitotic rate. Miettinen and colleagues[24]

have incorporated site of primary lesion (gastric versus small bowel) into a revised version of the risk assessment schema. This more recent risk assessment is now considered the standard risk assessment model.[25]

MOLECULAR BIOLOGY

Since the first discovery of activating *KIT* mutations by Hirota and colleagues, much progress has been made in the understanding and characterization of the various forms of *KIT* mutants. Eighty to 88% of GISTs are associated with a *KIT* mutation in either the exons 11, 9, 13, or 17. Exon 11 mutations are most common, occurring in approximately 65% of all cases, followed by exon 9 mutations (15%), with exon 13 and 17 representing approximately 1% of tumors each.[26–28] In 2002, Heinrich and co-workers reported an analogous gain-of-function mutation in a closely related receptor tyrosine kinase, platelet-derived growth factor receptor-α (PDGFRA), in approximately 35% of GISTs lacking *KIT* mutations. These *PDGFRA* mutant tumors were indistinguishable from *KIT* mutants with respect to activation of downstream signaling intermediates and cytogenetic changes related to tumor progression.[29] Based on this finding, subsequent mutational studies estimated frequency of *PDGFRA* mutations to be between 2% to 7%, and the remaining 7% to 13% of GISTs being wild-type for both *KIT* and *PDGFRA*. The significance of mutational status of GIST, as will be detailed later, lies in its correlation with clinical outcome in TKI treated patients.

Based on work by Corless and colleagues,[30] it is likely that activating *KIT* mutations are acquired early in the development of GISTs. In a cohort of 13 morphologically benign, small (4 mm–10 mm) asymptomatic GISTs identified incidentally, 11 samples harbored confirmed KIT mutations. In parallel to these findings, it is not unusual to find characteristics cytogenetic aberrations (deletions in 14q and 22q) in subsets of *KIT* mutant GISTs, but conversely some *KIT* mutant GISTs have entirely normal cytogenetic profiles. This would suggest that *KIT* activating mutations occur early in the course of disease but further chromosomal changes, including deletions in 14q, 22q, 1p, 11p and 9p, as well as gains in 8p and 17q, are necessary to effect overtly malignant phenotype and progression of disease.[31]

UNCOMMON PRESENTATIONS OF GIST
Pediatric GIST

Pediatric GIST is a rare childhood malignancy occurring preferentially in females. Evidence suggests that it may be biologically distinct from adult GISTs. Although pediatric GISTs express KIT at levels comparable to adult GISTs, fewer than 15% of tumors harbor activating *KIT* or *PDGFRA* mutations, in contrast to the more than 85% noted in adult GISTs. In addition, pediatric GISTs respond poorly to standard imatinib treatment, the cornerstone for adult GIST therapeutics. Interestingly, pediatric *KIT*-wild type GISTs display levels of KIT activation similar to that seen in both pediatric and adult *KIT*-mutant GISTs, suggesting that a separate biological mechanism may be responsible for its oncogenesis.[32] Recently, insulin-like growth factor-1 receptor (IGF-IR) amplification and protein expression has been detected in pediatric and wild-type GIST,[33,34] and is hypothesized to be associated with the oncogenesis of such tumors. This finding, if confirmed, may have therapeutic implications especially in the subset of tumors that respond poorly to imatinib-based therapy.

Familial GIST

Heritable mutations in *KIT* and *PDGFRA*, likely of autosomal dominant inheritance pattern, have been widely reported in the literature.[35–37] Affected kindreds with familial GIST may present with multi-focal disease, and in some cases, may be associated with cutaneous and mucous membrane hyperpigmentation, mast cell disease, urticaria pigmentosa and diffuse spindle cell hyperplasia in the myenteric plexus of the gastrointestinal tract. Carney's triad, a rare and possibly familial tumor syndrome, of unidentified genetic mechanism, predominantly affects young women, and comprises of gastric stromal sarcoma (GIST), pulmonary chondroma and extra-adrenal paraganglioma.[38] Neurofibromatosis type 1 has also been associated with development of GIST. In a Swedish population based study of 70 patients with NF-1, 7% of patients were diagnosed with GIST. These tumors are frequently multifocal, often affect the small bowel, and are often *KIT/PDGFRA* mutation negative.[39,40]

Treatment of Localized Disease

Standard treatment for localized, resectable GIST remains complete surgical resection. As GIST tends to be exophytic rather than diffusely infiltrative, wedge resection is oftentimes sufficient. In locations where wedge resection is not technically feasible, wide resection (esophagus GIST) and en-bloc (omental GIST) resections are recommended, aiming to achieve complete gross resection.[41] Lymphadenectomy is not warranted unless there is gross nodal involvement. In cases of unresectable or marginally resectable disease, neoadjuvant therapy with imatinib should be considered.[25,41]

The role of adjuvant imatinib therapy is being actively investigated. In the ACOSOG Z9000 trial, a United States intergroup phase 2 single-arm trial of adjuvant imatinib in patients with high-risk, completely resected GIST, one year of adjuvant imatinib prolonged recurrence-free survival compared with historical controls.[42] In a parallel phase 3 placebo-controlled study of adjuvant imatinib in patients with completely resected GIST, 3 cm or larger, ACOSOG Z9001, one-year of adjuvant imatinib significantly improved relapse-free survival compared with placebo, 97% 1-year relapse-free survival compared with 83% achieved with placebo. Notably, there was no significant difference in overall survival at a median follow-up of 15 months.[43]

Treatment of Advanced Disease

Before 2000, metastatic GIST was a uniformly fatal disease with few therapeutic options. Response to chemotherapy was invariably poor, with one study reporting an abysmal response rate of 1.8% despite aggressive combination chemotherapy.[44]

Imatinib is a small molecule tyrosine kinase inhibitor (TKI) with potent activity against the transmembrane receptor KIT, ABL kinase and chimeric BCR-ABL fusion oncoprotein product of chronic myeloid leukemia. Imatinib occupies the ATP binding pocket of KIT, thereby preventing substrate phosphorylation, downstream signaling and inhibiting cell proliferation and survival. Imatinib was first approved in 2002 for use in advanced GIST following impressive clinical activity demonstrated in a phase 2 study of 147 patients.[16] Overall, objective response rates of 53.7% and stable disease in 27.9% were achieved in this study population with very manageable toxicities. This represented a remarkable advancement in therapy for patients with metastatic GIST. With longer follow-up, these results continue to hold true. Overall median time to progression being 24 months and median overall survival reported as 57 months. Overall survival was not different in patients who achieved an objective response or stable disease.[45]

As the maximum tolerated dose of imatinib in a European phase 1 dose escalation study was 800 mg per day, there were concerns amongst GIST experts worldwide that patients might achieve greater benefit with higher dosing.[46] As such, two separate large phase 3 randomized studies were conducted on either side of the Atlantic, comparing imatinib 400 mg daily (standard dose) versus 800 mg daily, administered at 400 mg twice per day (high dose); crossover to the high-dose arm at time of disease progression was permitted for patients randomized to the standard dose.[47,48] Toxicities were greater in the high-dose arm, with more patients requiring dose reductions (16% in the standard arm versus 58%–60% in the high-dose arm) and dose interruptions (38%–40% in the standard arm versus 59%–64% in the high-dose arm). Common imatinib toxicities include edema, fatigue, nausea, rash and diarrhea. In a pooled analysis, a small but statistically significant progression-free survival (PFS) benefit was noted in the high-dose arm approximately 19 months versus 23 months, with results consistent in both studies (but significant only in the European study). For patients with KIT exon 9 mutation, PFS benefit was detected in the high-dose arm in the European study (19 months versus 4 months), not confirmed in the United States study, but nevertheless, remained significant in the pooled meta-analysis (19 months versus 6 months). There was no benefit seen for high-dose imatinib in patients with primary exon 11 mutations. Overall survival was identical in standard- and high-dose arms, independent of genotype.[49] Thus, a high-dose imatinib starting dose may reasonably improve PFS in patients with KIT exon 9 mutation, but is associated with greater toxicity, with no added survival benefit.

Sunitinib, a small molecule, oral, multitargeted tyrosine kinase inhibitor with potent anti-angiogenic and anti-tumor activities, targets receptors of KIT, vascular endothelial growth factor receptor (VEGF1, 2, 3), platelet-derived growth factor (PDGFA and B), Fms-like tyrosine kinase-3 (FLT3), and the receptor encoded by ret proto-oncogene (RET). Because of this broad spectrum of inhibition, sunitinib may have both antitumor and antiangiogenic effects in GIST. A randomized, placebo-controlled, multinational trial evaluated the benefit of sunitinib administered 50 mg daily, 4 weeks on and 2 weeks off. In this study, 312 patients with imatinib refractory or intolerant GIST were randomized in a 2:1 ratio to receive sunitinib (n = 207) or placebo (n = 105). The trial was unblinded early when an interim data analysis showed a significantly longer median time to progression (TTP) with sunitinib (6.8 months versus 1.6 months). The majority of patients on sunitinib (58%) achieved stable disease as their best response, with only 7% of patients demonstrating a partial response. Despite the cross over design of the trial, overall survival obtained with initial sunitinib was superior to that obtained with placebo (hazard ratio 0.49, P<.007). This pivotal study established the role of sunitinib as second- line therapy in patients with advanced imatinib-refractory or imatinib-intolerant GIST.[17]

Work by Van den Abbeele and colleagues,[50] using [18F] fluorodeoxyglucose-positron emission tomography (FDG PET) to study the effects of sunitinib on GIST, when administered on a 4-week on and 2-week off schedule, revealed that FDG responses were noted as early as 7 days. But this suppression was accompanied by a rebound during the 2- week off period, suggesting a flare in disease activity, consistent with lack of TK inhibition during the wash-out period. Thus, clinical studies employing continuous daily dosing of sunitinib have been undertaken in an attempt to provide consistent TK inhibition. Starting dose of sunitinib at 37.5 mg daily was chosen to reduce toxicity. In a report by George and colleagues,[51] continuous daily dosing was found to be safe and well tolerated. Median PFS of 32 weeks was achieved, comparable to results obtained from the 4-week on and 2-week off schedule. Longer follow-up for efficacy assessment is required.

Common sunitinib toxicities include fatigue, diarrhea, hand-foot syndrome, rash, and skin discoloration. Hypertension, likely a class effect of anti-angiogenic agents, is relatively common, and occurs in about 20% of treated patients, 5% being grade 3/4 in severity. Hypothyroidism, possibly secondary to a drug-related destructive thyroiditis process, via inhibition of the protein product of the RET proto-oncogene found on normal thyroid has been described in as high as 36% of sunitinib-treated GIST patients.[52] Cardiotoxicity has recently been reported to be associated with sunitinib use, although its frequency and significance varies considerably.[17,53]

FUTURE DIRECTIONS

Currently in ongoing trials, sorafenib tosylate, a small molecule Raf kinase and VEGF-receptor kinase inhibitor, has demonstrable activity in TKI-treated patients, yielding a 13% partial response rate in a group of 26 patients, 77% of whom were imatinib and sunitinib refractory. Progression-free survival and median overall survival are 5.3 months and 13 months respectively.[54] Heat shock proteins (HSP) control the proper folding, function, and stabilization of various "client" proteins. Many of these client proteins (eg, KIT and PDGFR-α) are oncoproteins or important cell signaling proteins. Inhibition of KIT signaling by targeting its molecular chaperone is an area of active research. Recently, IPI-504, a novel potent inhibitor of HSP-90, demonstrated clinical activity in a phase 1 dose escalation trial, achieving a 23% response rate (judged by positron emission tomography scans) and a median PFS of 12 weeks, in a cohort of heavily pretreated GIST patients.[55] At the time of this writing, an international phase 3 placebo-controlled study with IPI-504 in patients with imatinib and sunitinib refractory GIST is being planned. IGF-IR inhibitors are a new promising class of anti-cancer agents. In light of the finding of IGF-IR up-regulation in wild-type and pediatric GISTs, further studies are eagerly anticipated.

SUMMARY

The last decade marked an important era in the history of GIST, culminating from the discovery of near universal KIT protein expression and activating *KIT* mutations, in advancement of diagnosis of GIST and our understanding of its oncogenesis; to the development of risk stratification models, refining prognostication, and consequently, influencing treatment strategies; to the translation of laboratory successes into biologically relevant therapeutics, dramatically improving patient outcomes. It is with optimism that patients, clinicians, and researchers alike, stride into the next decade, working to improve on the remarkable achievements of the last.

REFERENCES

1. Stout AP. Bizarre smooth muscle tumors of the stomach. Cancer 1962;15:400.
2. Somerhausen Nde S, Fletcher CD. Gastrointestinal stromal tumours: an update. Sarcoma 1998;2(3-4):133–41.
3. Welsh RA, Meyer AT. Ultrastructure of gastric leiomyoma. Arch Pathol 1969;87(1): 71–81.
4. Weiss RA, Mackay B. Malignant smooth muscle tumors of the gastrointestinal tract: an ultrastructural study of 20 cases. Ultrastruct Pathol 1981;2(3):231–40.
5. Yagihashi S, Kimura M, Kurotaki H, et al. Gastric submucosal tumours of neurogenic origin with neuroaxonal and Schwann cell elements. J Pathol 1987; 153(1):41–50.

6. Mazur MT, Clark HB. Gastric stromal tumors. Reappraisal of histogenesis. Am J Surg Pathol 1983;7(6):507–19.

7. Herrera GA, Cerezo L, Jones JE, et al. Gastrointestinal autonomic nerve tumors. 'Plexosarcomas'. Arch Pathol Lab Med 1989;113(8):846–53.

8. Lauwers GY, Erlandson RA, Casper ES, et al. Gastrointestinal autonomic nerve tumors. A clinicopathological, immunohistochemical, and ultrastructural study of 12 cases. Am J Surg Pathol 1993;17(9):887–97.

9. Mikhael AI, Bacchi CE, Zarbo RJ, et al. CD34 expression in stromal tumors of the gastrointestinal tract. Appl Immunohistochem 1994;2:89–93.

10. Miettinen M, Virolainen M, Sarlomo-Rikala Maarit. Gastrointestinal stromal tumors-value of CD34 antigen in their identification and separation from true leiomyomas and schwannomas. Am J Surg Pathol 1995;19(2):207–16.

11. Nagata H, Worobec AS, Oh CK, et al. Identification of a point mutation in the catalytic domain of the proto-oncogene c-kit in peripheral blood mononuclear cells of patients who have mastocytosis with an associated hematologic disorder. Proc Natl Acad Sci U S A 1995;92(23):10560–4.

12. Longley BJ, Tyrrell L, Lu SZ, et al. Somatic c-KIT activating mutation in urticaria pigmentosa and aggressive mastocytosis: establishment of clonality in a human mast cell neoplasm. Nat Genet 1996;12(3):312–4.

13. Hirota S, Isozaki K, Moriyama Y, et al. Gain-of-function mutations of c-kit in human gastrointestinal stromal tumors. Science 1998;279(5350):577–80.

14. Kindblom LG, Remotti HE, Aldenborg F, et al. Gastrointestinal pacemaker cell tumor (GIPACT): gastrointestinal stromal tumors show phenotypic characteristics of the interstitial cells of Cajal. Am J Pathol 1998;152(5):1259–69.

15. Joensuu H, Roberts PJ, Sarlomo-Rikala M, et al. Effect of the tyrosine kinase inhibitor STI571 in a patient with a metastatic gastrointestinal stromal tumor. N Engl J Med 2001;344(14):1052–6.

16. Demetri GD, von Mehren M, Blanke CD, et al. Efficacy and safety of imatinib mesylate in advanced gastrointestinal stromal tumors. N Engl J Med 2002;347(7):472–80.

17. Demetri GD, van Oosterom AT, Garrett CR, et al. Efficacy and safety of sunitinib in patients with advanced gastrointestinal stromal tumour after failure of imatinib: a randomised controlled trial. Lancet 2006;368(9544):1329–38.

18. DeMatteo RP, Lewis JJ, Leung D, et al. Two hundred gastrointestinal stromal tumors: recurrence patterns and prognostic factors for survival. Ann Surg 2000;231(1):51–8.

19. Joensuu H, Fletcher C, Dimitrijevic S, et al. Management of malignant gastrointestinal stromal tumours. Lancet Oncol 2002;3(11):655–64.

20. Nilsson B, Bümming P, Meis-Kindblom JM, et al. Gastrointestinal stromal tumors: the incidence, prevalence, clinical course, and prognostication in the preimatinib mesylate era- a population-based study in western Sweden. Cancer 2005;103(4): 821–9.

21. Fletcher CD, Berman JJ, Corless C, et al. Diagnosis of gastrointestinal stromal tumors: a consensus approach. Hum Pathol 2002;33(5):459–65.

22. Rudolph P, Gloeckner K, Parwaresch R, et al. Immunophenotype, proliferation, DNA ploidy, and biological behavior of gastrointestinal stromal tumors: a multivariate clinicopathologic study. Hum Pathol 1998;29(8):791–800.

23. Emory TS, Sobin LH, Lukes L, et al. Prognosis of gastrointestinal smooth-muscle (stromal) tumors: dependence on anatomic site. Am J Surg Pathol 1999;23(1): 82–7.

24. Miettinen M, Lasota J. Gastrointestinal stromal tumors: pathology and prognosis at different sites. Semin Diagn Pathol 2006;23(2):70–83.

25. Demetri GD, Benjamin RS, Blanke CD, et al. NCCN Task Force report: management of patients with gastrointestinal stromal tumor (GIST)- update of the NCCN clinical practice guidelines. J Natl Compr Canc Netw 2007;5(Suppl 2):S1–29.
26. Heinrich MC, Corless CL, Demetri GD, et al. Kinase mutations and imatinib response in patients with metastatic gastrointestinal stromal tumor. J Clin Oncol 2003;21(23):4342–9.
27. Corless CL, Fletcher JA, Heinrich MC. Biology of gastrointestinal stromal tumors. J Clin Oncol 2004;22(18):3813–25.
28. Debiec-Rychter M, Sciot R, Le Cesne A, et al. KIT mutations and dose selection for imatinib in patients with advanced gastrointestinal stromal tumours. Eur J Cancer 2006;42(8):1093–103.
29. Heinrich MC, Corless CL, Duensing A, et al. PDGFRA activating mutations in gastrointestinal stromal tumors. Science 2003;299(5607):708–10.
30. Corless CL, McGreevey L, Haley A, et al. KIT mutations are common in incidental gastrointestinal stromal tumors one centimeter or less in size. Am J Pathol 2002; 160(5):1567–72.
31. Heinrich MC, Rubin BP, Longley BJ, et al. Biology and genetic aspects of gastrointestinal stromal tumors: KIT activation and cytogenetic alterations. Hum Pathol 2002;33(5):484–95.
32. Janeway KA, Liegl B, Harlow A, et al. Pediatric KIT wild-type and platelet-derived growth factor receptor alpha-wild-type gastrointestinal stromal tumors share KIT activation but not mechanisms of genetic progression with adult gastrointestinal stromal tumors. Cancer Res 2007;67(19):9084–8.
33. Agaram NP, Laquaglia MP, Ustun B, et al. Molecular characterization of pediatric gastrointestinal stromal tumors. Clin Cancer Res 2008;14(10):3204–15.
34. Tarn C, Rink L, Merkel E, et al. Insulin-like growth factor 1 receptor is a potential therapeutic target for gastrointestinal stromal tumors. Proc Natl Acad Sci U S A 2008;105(24):8387–92.
35. Kleinbaum EP, Lazar AJ, Tamborini E, et al. Clinical, histopathologic, molecular and therapeutic findings in a large kindred with gastrointestinal stromal tumor. Int J Cancer 2008;122(3):711–8.
36. Li FP, Fletcher JA, Heinrich MC, et al. Familial gastrointestinal stromal tumor syndrome: phenotypic and molecular features in a kindred. J Clin Oncol 2005; 23(12):2735–43.
37. Chompret A, Kannengiesser C, Barrois M, et al. PDGFRA germline mutation in a family with multiple cases of gastrointestinal stromal tumor. Gastroenterology 2004;126(1):318–21.
38. Carney JA. Gastric stromal sarcoma, pulmonary chondroma, and extra-adrenal paraganglioma (Carney Triad): natural history, adrenocortical component, and possible familial occurrence. Mayo Clin Proc 1999;74(6):543–52.
39. Zöller ME, Rembeck B, Odén A, et al. Malignant and benign tumors in patients with neurofibromatosis type 1 in a defined Swedish population. Cancer 1997; 79(11):2125–31.
40. Miettinen M, Fetsch JF, Sobin LH, et al. Gastrointestinal stromal tumors in patients with neurofibromatosis 1: a clinicopathologic and molecular genetic study of 45 cases. Am J Surg Pathol 2006;30(1):90–6.
41. Blay JY, Bonvalot S, Casali P, et al. Consensus meeting for the management of gastrointestinal stromal tumors. Report of the GIST Consensus Conference of 20-21 March 2004, under the auspices of ESMO. Ann Oncol 2005;16(4):566–78.
42. DeMatteo RP, Owzar K, Antonescu CR, et al. Efficacy of adjuvant imatinib mesylate following complete resection of localized, primary gastrointestinal stromal

tumor (GIST) at high risk of recurrence: The U.S. Intergroup phase II trial ACOSOG Z9000. J Clin Oncol 2005;23(16S):9009.

43. DeMatteo RP, Owzar K, Maki R, et al. Adjuvant imatinib mesylate increases recurrence free survival (RFS) in patients with completely resected localized primary gastrointestinal stromal tumor (GIST): North American Intergroup Phase III trial ACOSOG Z9001. 2005 American Society of Clinical Oncology Annual Meeting Proceedings, Orlando, FL, May 13–17, 2005.

44. Edmonson JH, Marks RS, Buckner JC, et al. Contrast of response to dacarbazine, mitomycin, doxorubicin, and cisplatin (DMAP) plus GM-CSF between patients with advanced malignant gastrointestinal stromal tumors and patients with other advanced leiomyosarcomas. Cancer Invest 2002;20(5-6):605–12.

45. Blanke CD, Demetri GD, von Mehren M, et al. Long-term results from a randomized phase II trial of standard- versus higher-dose imatinib mesylate for patients with unresectable or metastatic gastrointestinal stromal tumors expressing KIT. J Clin Oncol 2008;26(4):620–5.

46. Van Oosterom AT, Judson I, Verweij J, et al. Safety and efficacy of imatinib (STI571) in metastatic gastrointestinal stromal tumours: a phase I study. Lancet 2001;358(9291):1421–3.

47. Blanke CD, Rankin C, Demetri GD, et al. Phase III randomized, intergroup trial assessing imatinib mesylate at two dose levels in patients with unresectable or metastatic gastrointestinal stromal tumors expressing the kit receptor tyrosine kinase: S0033. J Clin Oncol 2008;26(4):626–32.

48. Verweij J, Casali PG, Zalcberg J, et al. Progression-free survival in gastrointestinal stromal tumours with high-dose imatinib: randomised trial. Lancet 2004; 364(9440):1127–34.

49. Van Glabbeke MM, Owzar K, Rankin C, et al. Comparison of two doses of imatinib for the treatment of unresectable or metastatic gastrointestinal stromal tumors (GIST): a meta-analyis based on 1,640 patients (pts). J Clin Oncol 2007; 25(18S):10004.

50. Van den Abbeele A, Melenevsky Y, de Vries D, et al. Imaging kinase target inhibition with SU11248 by FDG-PET in patients (pts) with imatinib-resistant gastrointestinal stromal tumors (I-R GIST). J Clin Oncol 2005;23(16S):9006.

51. George S, Blay JY, Casali PG, et al. Continuous daily dosing (CDD) of sunitinib (SU) in pts with advanced GIST: updated efficacy, safety, PK and pharmacodynamic analysis. J Clin Oncol 2008;26 [May 20 suppl; abstr 10554].

52. Desai J, Yassa L, Marqusee E, et al. Hypothyroidism after sunitinib treatment for patients with gastrointestinal stromal tumors. Ann Intern Med 2006;145(9):660–4.

53. Chu TF, Rupnick MA, Kerkela R, et al. Cardiotoxicity associated with tyrosine kinase inhibitor sunitinib. Lancet 2007;370(9604):2011–9.

54. Wiebe L, Kasza KE, Maki RG, et al. Activity of sorafenib (SOR) in patients (pts) with imatinib (IM) and sunitinib (SU)-resistant (RES) gastrointestinal stromal tumors (GIST): a phase II trial of the University of Chicago Phase II Consortium. J Clin Oncol 2008;26 [May 20 suppl; abstr 10502].

55. Wagner AJ, Morgan JA, Chugh R, et al. Inhibition of heat shock protein 90 (Hsp90) with the novel agent IPI-504 in metastatic GIST following failure of tyrosine kinase inhibitors (TKIs) or other sarcomas: clinical results from phase I trial. J Clin Oncol 2008;26 [May 20 suppl; abstr 10502].

Management of Resectable Gastrointestinal Stromal Tumor

Umer I. Chaudhry, MD, Ronald P. DeMatteo, MD*

KEYWORDS

- Gastrointestinal stromal tumor • KIT • PDGFR • Mutation
- Surgery

The literature on gastrointestinal stromal tumors (GISTs) has expanded exponentially, demonstrating how medical advancement in the understanding of a disease can revolutionize its diagnosis and treatment. In the past, these tumors were classified as leiomyomas, leiomyosarcomas, or leiomyoblastomas. Only recently has it become evident that GIST is a separate entity and the most common sarcoma of the gastrointestinal (GI) tract.[1,2]

GIST is a mesenchymal tumor that mainly arises from the alimentary tract but also can develop in the omentum and mesentery. The term GIST first was coined in 1983 by Mazur and Clark to describe GI nonepithelial neoplasms that lacked immunohistochemical features of Schwann cells, and did not encompass ultrastructural characteristics of smooth muscle cells.[1] GISTs continued to be diagnosed rarely until late 1990s, when they became a focus of intense investigation. In 1998, Hirota and colleagues[3] reported that most GISTs harbored gain-of-function mutations in the KIT (also called CD117) proto-oncogene, a hallmark of GIST.

The KIT gene encodes the KIT protein, which serves as the transmembrane receptor for the cytokine known as stem cell factor (SCF). The intracytoplasmic portion of KIT functions as a tyrosine kinase.[4] Subsequent reports have found KIT mutations in up to 85% of GISTs, while another 3% to 5% GISTs harbor platelet-derived growth factor receptor α (PDGFRα) mutations.[5–7] PDGFRα also exhibits tyrosine kinase function.

In 2001, Joensuu and colleagues[8] discovered imatinib mesylate to be highly effective against chemotherapy-resistant GIST. Imatinib is a molecular inhibitor of the KIT

Ronald P. DeMatteo is a consultant to and on the advisory board of Novartis. He is also a speaker for and has received honoraria from Novartis.
Hepatobiliary Service, Memorial Sloan-Kettering Cancer Center, Box 203, 1275 York Avenue, New York, NY 10021, USA
* Corresponding author.
E-mail address: dematter@mskcc.org (R.P. DeMatteo).

and PDGFRα proteins. The dramatic response achieved in a solid tumor with targeted agent imatinib has made GIST a paradigm for the use of new molecular agents. Over 80% of patients benefit from tyrosine kinase inhibitor therapy, and median survival from the diagnosis of metastatic GIST is now nearly 5 years.[9,10]

EPIDEMIOLOGY

GISTs demonstrate a fairly equal distribution between men and woman, although some literature suggests that GIST has a slight male predominance.[10] The precise incidence of GIST in the United States is difficult to quantify because of its recent identification as a separate entity. The Surveillance, Epidemiology, and End Results (SEER) program of National Cancer Institute's (NCI) report in 1995 indicated 500 to 600 new cases of GIST were diagnosed in the United States annually.[11] Recent guidelines published by National Comprehensive Cancer Network (NCCN) estimate the incidence of GIST in the United States to be near 5000.[12,13] Furthermore, based on a recent study from Sweden, the estimated annual incidence of GIST in the United States similarly would be 4000 to 5000.[14] As clinicians become more acquainted with the molecular, histologic, and clinical features of this disease, there will be a better understanding of the true incidence and prevalence of GIST. Although GIST has been documented in patients of all ages, most of the people affected by GIST are between 40 and 80 years old at the time of diagnosis, with the median age of 60 years.[10]

Most GISTs are sporadic. There are a few case reports, however, of familial germline mutations in the KIT proto-oncogene, and one family carried a PDGFRα mutation.[15,16] Additionally, GIST has been diagnosed in hereditary syndromes such as neurofibromatosis[17] and Carney's traid,[18] a rare entity that predominantly occurs in young women and is associated with gastric GIST, paraganglioma, and pulmonary chondroma. Only 25% of the patients, however, manifest the complete triad. Approximately 60% of GISTs occur in the stomach, 30% in the small intestine, 5% in the rectum, and 5% in the esophagus.[10,19] Rarely, GIST may develop outside of the alimentary tract in locations such as the mesentery, omentum, pancreas, or other retroperitoneal structures.[20] Although GIST is the most common mesenchymal tumor in the GI tract, leiomyomas predominate in the esophagus.[21]

As mentioned previously, although GIST predominates in adults over 40 years of age, it also can occur in children and younger adults, with unique clincopathologic distinctions. Children are more likely to present with multifocal gastric tumors, harbor epithelioid histology, contain wild-type KIT/PDGFRα genome, and possess a higher rate of lymph node (LN) metastasis.[22] In young adult patients, GISTs can present either as the pediatric- or adult-type tumors. The unique gene expression profile of GIST in the pediatric and young adult population is an intensive area of investigation, to gain a finer understanding of the complex pathophysiology of the disease.

HISTOPATHOLOGY

The histopathologic diagnosis of GIST has had significant advancement over the last several years, mainly as a result of the recent progress in the understanding of molecular pathogenesis of GIST. Demonstrating characteristics of smooth muscle cells under microscopy, these unique tumors initially were characterized as leiomyomas when exhibiting benign features and leiomyosarcoma when displaying malignant characteristics.[23,24] Advances in medicine and technology led to identification of cellular features in GISTs, which were consistent with neural elements.[25] Soon, it was found that most GISTs express CD117 or KIT, a transmembrane growth factor receptor with tyrosine kinase activity,[3] and arise from a KIT-positive interstitial cell of Cajal

(ICC), the pacemaker cell of the GI tract.[26] Normally, KIT is found in its inactive confirmation. When bound by its ligand, however, KIT activates various other kinases including MAP kinase, STAT5, RAS, JAK2, and PI3 kinase, leading to cellular proliferation, differentiation, and adhesion.[27] Although up to 85% of GISTs express the KIT mutation, another 3% to 5% possess a PDGFRα mutation, and 10% to 15% of the cases contain the wild-type forms of these proto-oncogenes, yet overexpress KIT.[5–7] Activating KIT mutations, similar to those described in GISTs, were reported recently in a subset of acral and mucosal malignant melanomas.[28]

Histologically, GISTs can be characterized as spindle cell type (70%), epithelioid type (20%), or a rare mixed type where both features are present.[29] Spindle cell GISTs appear as uniform fusiform cells in intersecting fascicles or whorls. Epithelioid GISTs typically appear as rounded cells in a nested pattern. GISTs usually have scant stroma and uniform cytology with fibrillary eosinophilic cytoplasm and nuclei containing fine chromatin and inconspicuous nucleoli (**Fig. 1**).[30]

Although expressing KIT (CD117), GISTs may be positive for CD34 (60% to 70%) or smooth-muscle actin (SMA; 30% to 40%), and approximately 5% stain positive for S-100 protein.[31] GISTs rarely express desmin, but when desmin is found, it is invariably focal, with only small numbers of immunopositive cells. The diagnosis of KIT-negative GIST can present difficulty and depends on tissue morphology and genotyping the tumor for a KIT or PDGFRα mutation, as some tumors negative for KIT by immunohistochemistry have mutations in either of the proto-oncogenes.[32,33]

Unlike other GI malignancies, the behavior of GIST is difficult to predict based on histopathology alone. The best indicator of malignancy is the confirmation of metastatic disease. The three most important characteristics that have shown some ability to predict how GISTs will behave are size, mitotic rate, and location of tumor.[34] Tumors with low mitotic counts (less than 5 per 50 high power field [HPF]) and diameters less than 2 cm generally exhibit benign behavior, while diameters greater than 10 cm and high mitotic counts (more than 5 per 50 HPF) are associated with malignant behavior. Tumors located in the stomach have a more favorable outcome. Importantly, neither small size nor low mitotic rate excludes the potential for malignant behavior.[35,36]

H&E	CD117 (KIT)

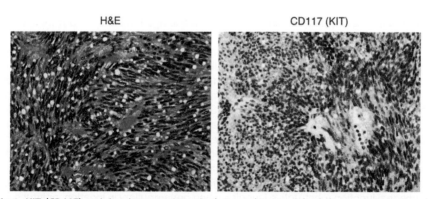

Fig. 1. KIT (CD117) staining in gastrointestinal stromal tumor. The left panel shows hematoxylin and eosin staining, and the right panel demonstrates KIT immunohistochemistry of the same tumor. Diffuse, high-level KIT staining is typical. Magnification 40×. (*Courtesy of* Dr. Cristina Antonescu, Department of Pathology, Memorial Sloan-Kettering Cancer Center.)

MOLECULAR GENETICS

The KIT proto-oncogene is found on chromosome 4q11-q12 and controls KIT expression. KIT is expressed by ICCs, which are the pacemaker cells of the alimentary tract and believed to give rise to GISTs. Additionally, KIT is found in hematopoietic cells, mast cells, and germ cells. The natural ligand for KIT has several names, including KIT ligand, SCF, steel factor, and mast cell growth factor. KIT is involved in many cellular functions, including differentiation, cell growth, and survival. Binding of KIT to its ligand leads to dimerization and autophosphorylation of KIT, which initiates a cascade of intracellular signaling, leading to adhesion, differentiation, proliferation, and tumorigenesis. In GIST, a gain-of-function mutation in KIT leads to constitutive activation of KIT and its tyrosine kinase function.[3] In a transgenic mouse model, KIT mutation has been shown to be sufficient in inducing GIST formation.[37] Several other malignancies including mastocytosis,[38] germ cell tumors,[39] acute myelogenous leukemia,[40] and neuroblastoma[41] also have been shown to express activating KIT mutations.

KIT mutation can occur in up to 85% of GISTs and is nearly always somatic.[5] Various forms of KIT mutations have been detected in GISTs. The most common sites involve KIT exon 11 (70% of GISTs), whereas an exon 9 mutation occurs in approximately 10% of cases. Mutations of exon 13 or 17 are found rarely.[5,6,42] Approximately 3% to 5% of GISTs harbor mutations in exons 12, 14, and 18 of PDGFRα proto-oncogene.[43] Interestingly, about 10% to 15% of the patients who have GISTs do not possess a detectable mutation in either of the two proto-oncogenes. At the level of the chromosomes, there have been other abnormalities confirmed in the development of GIST, such as early loss of 14p and 22q, which may suggest that chromosomal derangement may represent another mechanism for cancer progression.[44] Approximately 3% of GISTs are found in the pediatric population.[22]

PRESENTATION AND DIAGNOSIS

Although almost 70% of patients who harbor GIST suffer from vague symptoms, the diagnosis often is made only after laparotomy for other pathology and detailed pathologic examination. Because of the scarcity of this tumor, the disease rarely is suspected before the time of surgery. Preoperative diagnosis of GIST requires a high degree of suspicion, and certain key radiologic findings may hint toward the elusive diagnosis.[45]

The most common presenting symptoms of GISTs are GI bleeding, abdominal discomfort, and abdominal mass. These all likely result from the fact that GISTs are fast-growing tumors that quickly outgrow their blood supply. As a result, they develop a necrotic center (evident on radiologic imaging), which can fistulize to an enteric lumen and result in GI bleeding. Rarely, GISTs can rupture into the abdominal cavity and cause massive intraperitoneal hemorrhage. Because GISTs tend to displace adjacent organs rather than invade them, they may become quite large before causing symptoms such as nausea, emesis, bloating, early satiety, increased abdominal girth or a palpable mass, which are all nonspecific. As with other neoplasms that arise in certain locations, GISTs can cause dysphagia when found in the esophagus or gastro-esophageal junction, obstructive jaundice when periampullary in location, or intussusception with obstruction in the small bowel.[45,46] A recent population-based study demonstrated that approximately 70% of GISTs induce symptoms, while 20% do not cause any symptoms, and 10% are detected at time of autopsy. The median tumor size for these categories was 8.9 cm, 2.7 cm, and 3.4 cm, respectively.[14]

GISTs are diagnosed most frequently during workup for other pathology. Depending on their location, they may be identified as masses on esophagogastroduodenoscopy, colonoscopy, CT, or MRI. The most useful radiologic study for the diagnosis of GISTs is the CT scan. Contrast-enhanced CT can evaluate the primary tumor and the liver and peritoneum, which are the most common sites metastatic disease. Lymph node metastases are extremely rare. Metastases in the lungs and other extra-abdominal locations usually are observed only in advanced cases. A primary tumor is typically a well-circumscribed and often highly vascular mass closely associated with the stomach or small intestine. GISTs may appear heterogeneous because of central necrosis or intratumoral hemorrhage. On CT, GISTs usually appear as hyperdense, enhancing masses. Unfortunately, neither CT nor MRI can predict accurately whether the tumor has invaded adjacent structures. Fluorodeoxyglucose positron emission tomography (^{18}FDG-PET) has been shown to be sensitive in identifying metabolic activity within these tumors, but it is not specific enough for the diagnosis of GIST. PET, however, is useful at present in determining the clinical response to molecular treatment of GISTs (**Fig. 2**).[45]

Endoscopy may lead to diagnosis of gastric or colorectal GIST. On endoscopic evaluation, GIST appears as a submucosal mass. Endoscopic ultrasound can be useful to confirm that a tumor originates from the bowel wall and not the mucosa. As GISTs rarely initially metastasize to the chest, a chest radiograph is appropriate

Pre-Treatment   Post-Treatment

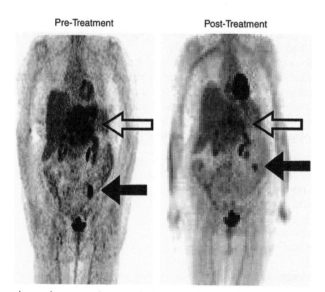

Fig. 2. ^{18} Fluorodeoxyglucose positron emission tomography FDG-PET scan showing response of metastatic gastrointestinal stromal tumor to imatinib mesylate. The patient presented with synchronous primary disease in the small bowel and metastatic disease in the liver. The scan on the left was obtained at presentation, and the scan on the right was obtained after 3 weeks of therapy. In the interval, there has been a decrease in size and ^{18}FDG uptake in both the small bowel and liver tumors consistent with a good response to imatinib. The standardized uptake value (SUV) of the liver metastases, shown with the open arrow, went from SUV 10.6 to 4.6, whereas the SUV of the primary tumor, shown with the closed arrow, went from 11 to 4.3. The patient eventually went on to complete surgical resection. (*From* Gold JS, DeMatteo RP. Combined surgical and molecular therapy: the gastrointestinal stromal tumor model. Ann Surg 2006;244:176; with permission.)

to assess the thorax. Bone scan should be ordered only to work-up specific symptoms. Percutaneous biopsy rarely should be used to confirm the diagnosis of a resectable GIST, as it can precipitate tumor rupture and lead to tumor dissemination or hemorrhage. Additionally, it may be extremely challenging to diagnose GIST from a percutaneous biopsy (fine needle aspiration or core needle) if necrotic or hemorrhagic tissue is sampled. Percutaneous biopsy is indicated if the results will change the management. For instance, if another diagnosis is entertained, such as a lymphoma, then the patient may not benefit from surgical resection. A biopsy also may be helpful in cases where the mass is marginally resectable, and neoadjuvant molecular treatment is desirable.

GISTs manifest a spectrum of clinical behavior. It is difficult to predict whether any particular GIST will recur after complete resection. Several variables have been identified to predict the clinical behavior of GIST. Tumor size, mitotic index, and tumor location are the three most important prognostic variables for GIST.[19,47] In a recent multivariate analysis from Memorial Sloan-Kettering Cancer Center,[34] each of these variables was found to independently predict recurrence-free survival after excision of primary, localized GIST (**Fig. 3**). The effect of mitotic rate was the most dramatic, with a hazard ratio (HR) of 14.6 for patients with at least 5 mitoses per 50 HPF (see **Fig. 3**C). Patients who had tumors located in small bowel (see **Fig. 3**A) and tumors at least 10 cm in size (see **Fig. 3**B) were also more likely to recur, with HR of 3.3 and 2.5, respectively. Patients with tumor size less than 5 cm or tumor located in the stomach had more favorable outcomes. Upon univariate analysis, patients who had KIT exon 9 mutations or KIT exon 11 deletions involving amino acid W557 and/ or K558 had a higher rate of recurrence (see **Fig. 3**D). Point mutations and insertions of KIT exon 11 had a favorable prognosis.

In addition to tumor size, mitotic rate, and location, several other variables have been investigated in their ability to predict recurrence.[47] Although complete gross resection has been associated with improved outcome,[48] so far microscopically positive margins have not been shown to impact survival (**Fig. 4**).[10] Tumor rupture either before or during resection has been correlated with poor outcome and often leads to peritoneal metastasis.[49] Prognostic factors for GIST include:

Tumor size
Mitotic rate
Location of primary tumor
Completeness of resection
Tumor rupture
Cellular proliferation index (Ki67)
Diffuse mucosal invasion
Aneuploidy
Telomerase expression
Extent of disease

Cellular proliferation estimated by Ki67 immunohistochemistry has been shown to be an independent prognostic factor.[50] Diffuse mucosal invasion is a rare finding and associated with an aggressive disease course.[51] Aneuploidy is a marker of malignancy,[50,52,53] and several studies have suggested telomerase expression as a poor prognostic factor.[49,54] KIT immunoreactivity or staining pattern and CD34 expression do not appear to be independent prognostic factors for survival.[43]

Despite these established prognostic factors, predicting clinical behavior of a GIST in a particular patient remains a challenge. It is accepted that all GISTs can exhibit malignant potential and none, except perhaps less than 1 cm tumors, can be labeled

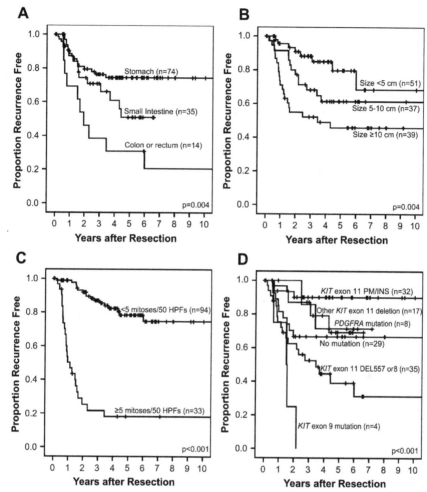

Fig. 3. (*A*) Recurrence-free survival in 127 patients with completely resected localized gastrointestinal stromal tumor based on tumor location, (*B*) tumor size, (*C*) mitotic rate, (*D*) and the type of mutation. (*From* DeMatteo RP, Gold JS, Saran L, et al. Tumor mitotic rate, size, and location independently predict recurrence after resection of primary gastrointestinal stromal tumor (GIST). Cancer 2008;112(3):608; with permission.)

as definitely benign.[45] Therefore, most pathologists classify GISTs as having very low, low, intermediate, or high risk for malignancy.[54] There are general guidelines established to group GISTs into one of these risk categories (**Table 1**).[4,29,35,47] Tumors greater than 5 to 10 cm in size and containing more than 5 mitoses per 50 HPFs are considered high risk for malignancy. It should be made clear, however, that even GISTs with low mitotic index (less than 5 mitoses per 50 HPFs) may possess malignant potential.[55] Between 10% and 25% of patients present with metastatic disease.[56]

Historically, patients who underwent complete surgical resection had a local recurrence rate of approximately 50%, with median time to recurrence of 24 months.[10,57] Recurrence tends to involve the peritoneal surface, the liver, or both. The authors found liver to be involved in 63% of the 80 patients who underwent complete resection of their primary tumor, and it was the only site of recurrence in 44% of the

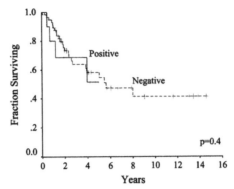

Fig. 4. Disease-specific survival by margin status in patients with primary disease who underwent complete resection (n = 80). (*From* DeMatteo RP, Lewis JJ, Leung D, et al. Two hundred gastrointestinal stromal tumors: recurrence patterns and prognostic factors for survival. Ann Surg 2000;231:51; with permission.)

recurrences.[10] Similarly, a study from the M.D. Anderson Cancer Center showed that nearly 40% of patients had recurrence confined to the peritoneum.[57] There may be a benefit to resecting recurrent isolated local or metastatic disease in highly selected patients when all gross tumor can be removed,[58] as the typical pattern of disease at the time of death is overwhelming intraperitoneal or intrahepatic tumor burden.

TREATMENT
Primary Disease

For patients who have primary localized GIST, surgical resection remains the only chance for cure.[59] It typically carries little morbidity for tumors less than 10 cm that are confined to the stomach or small intestine. Resection usually can be accomplished with wedge resection of the stomach or a segmental resection of the small bowel. Extensive surgery rarely is required. Every effort should be spent to obtain gross negative margins, but wide margins have not been associated with better prognosis (see **Fig. 4**),[10] as GIST does not exhibit an intramural spreading behavior. Because GISTs rarely metastasize to lymph nodes, formal lymphadenectomy is not necessary unless locoregional lymph nodes are enlarged. When adherence to adjacent organs is identified, an en bloc resection is favored. An incomplete resection should be only performed as a palliative therapy for bleeding, pain, or symptoms secondary to mass effect. Complete gross resection is possible in 85% of patients who have primary,

Table 1		
Assessment of the risk of recurrence in respectable gastrointestinal stromal tumor		
Risk Category	**Size**	**Mitotic Count**
Very low risk	<2 cm	<5/50 HPF
Low risk	2–5 cm	<5/50 HPF
Intermediate risk	<5 cm 5–10 cm	6–10/50 HPF <5/50 HPF
High risk	>10 cm any size >5 cm	Any mitotic rate >10/50 HPF >5/50 HPF

Abbreviation: HPF, high power field.
  Data from Fletcher CD, Berman JJ, Corless C, et al. Diagnosis of gastrointestinal stromal tumors: a consensus approach. Hum Pathol 2002;33(5):459–65.

localized disease. Nevertheless, historically, at least 50% of patients developed tumor recurrence, and 5-year survival was approximately 50% (**Fig. 5**).[10,49]

Conventional chemotherapy for the treatment of GIST has a dismal response rate of approximately 5%.[60–63] Radiotherapy is also of limited value, owing to the location of the tumors and the limit this places on the doses that can be employed.[43] Additionally, treatments such as hepatic artery embolization and debulking surgery followed by intraperitoneal chemotherapy have been investigated but with discouraging results.[64]

The development of imatinib mesylate has revolutionized the treatment of GISTs. Imatinib is a selective inhibitor of specific tyrosine kinases, including KIT, PDGFRα, ARG, c-FMS, ABL, and BCR-ABL.[65] Imatinib initially was developed as a PDGFRα inhibitor. Its first use as a therapeutic agent was for treating chronic myeloid leukemia (CML), in which a BCR-ABL fusion protein leads to an unregulated tyrosine kinase activity.[66] Imatinib has been shown to induce a complete response in nearly all patients in the chronic phase of CML.

In 2001, Joensuu and colleagues[8] published their experience with the treatment of metastatic GIST in a single patient with imatinib. The results were dramatic as seen on serial MRI and PET imaging. This landmark case report prompted several clinical trials, and it is now apparent that up to 80% of patients who have metastatic GIST achieve partial response or remain with stable disease while on imatinib.[30] Imatinib usually is tolerated well, and the adverse effect profile includes edema, rash, diarrhea, nausea, abdominal pain, and fatigue.

The use of adjuvant imatinib after complete resection of primary GIST was evaluated in a phase 2 trial led by the American College of Surgeons Oncology Group (ACOSOG), and sponsored by the Cancer Therapy Evaluation Program (CTEP) and Novartis. The study aimed to answer whether adjuvant imatinib at a dose of 400 mg/d for 12 months after complete resection of the primary tumor in high-risk patients can lead to decreased recurrence rates and improved 3-year survival. High risk was defined as a tumor size greater than 10 cm, intraperitoneal tumor rupture or hemorrhage, or multifocal (more than five) tumors. There were 107 evaluable patients enrolled between September 2001 and September 2003. Imatinib was initiated at a median of 59 (range 25 to 84) days after operation. The median age was 58 years (range 19 to 79). The median tumor size was 13 cm (range 3 to 42), and 50% of tumors originated from the stomach, while 42% arose in the small intestine. At a median

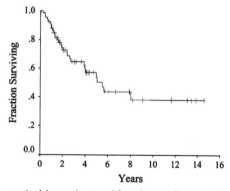

Fig. 5. Disease-specific survival in patients with primary disease who underwent complete resection (n = 80). (*From* DeMatteo RP, Lewis JJ, Leung D, et al. Two hundred gastrointestinal stromal tumors: recurrence patterns and prognostic factors for survival. Ann Surg 2000;231:51; with permission.)

follow-up of 4 years, the 1-, 2-, and 3-year overall survival rates were 99%, 97%, and 97%, respectively. The 1-, 2-, and 3-year recurrence-free survival rates were 94%, 73%, and 61%, respectively. The data from this trial have shown that imatinib is tolerated well in the adjuvant setting, prolongs recurrence-free survival, and is associated with improved overall survival when compared with historical controls.[67] There were no common terminology criteria grade 4 or grade 5 toxicities reported; 18% of patients had grade 3 adverse events, and 83% of the patients completed the 12 months of imatinib therapy.[68] Additionally, a randomized, double-blinded phase 3 ACOSOG intergroup trial in which patients received imatinib (400 mg/d) or placebo for 1 year after undergoing complete resection of their primary GIST (at least 3 cm tumor size) has just been completed. Accrual to the trial was halted because of a recommendation of the ACOSOG External Data Monitoring Committee based on the results of a planned interim analysis of 644 evaluable patients. Median follow-up time in recurrence-free patients was 1.2 years; 21% of the expected events had occurred. Patients assigned to the imatinib arm had a 1-year recurrence-free survival of 97%, while those assigned to the placebo arm had a 1-year recurrence-free survival of 83%, with a hazard ratio of 0.325 (95% CI 0.198 to 0.534), and a nominal unadjusted log-rank p-value of 0.0000014. No difference in overall survival between the two treatment arms was noted. Measuring overall survival, however, is immature at the time of this publication. Patients will continue to be followed per protocol, for up to 10 years. These original results support the role of imatinib in the adjuvant setting.[69] A phase 2 neoadjuvant trial for primary GIST led by the Radiation Therapy Oncology Group (RTOG) also has met accrual, and will define the role of imatinib in a preoperative setting. Neoadjuvant imatinib is particularly attractive for patient populations with large or poorly localized tumors that otherwise would require extensive surgery or sacrifice large amounts of normal tissue. Neoadjuvant therapy may convert the resection of a rectal GIST from an abdominoperineal resection to a low anterior resection. It should be mentioned that positive KIT staining on immunohistochemistry is an inclusion criterion for all these trials.

As there is effective treatment for recurrent or metastatic GIST, the NCCN recommends CT scans of the abdomen and pelvis with intravenous contrast every 3 to 6 months during the first 3 to 5 postoperative years and yearly thereafter.[13]

Recurrent and Metastatic Disease

In patients for whom curative surgery is not feasible, or who develop recurrent metastatic disease, imatinib is the first line treatment.[9,70] In fact, most patients will present with tumor recurrence despite undergoing complete resection of their primary tumor.[10] The median time to recurrence is reported to range from 18 to 24 months. At the time of recurrence, approximately two thirds of the patients have liver involvement, and half present with peritoneal disease.[10] Extra-abdominal metastasis to lung or bone may develop as the disease progresses.

Surgery alone has limited efficacy in recurrent or metastatic GIST. Excision of peritoneal disease usually is followed by subsequent recurrence. Liver metastases are usually multifocal, but approximately 26% of the patients remain candidates for resection.[63] Essentially all of the patients, however, develop recurrent disease after hepatic resection.

The gold standard for treatment of recurrent metastatic GIST is imatinib, with few exceptions. Patients who have primary GIST with synchronous, low-volume metastatic disease may be considered for surgical resection first, especially if they are symptomatic. Imatinib is reported to produce a partial tumor response in 45% of patients and stable disease in approximately 30%. Remarkably, the 2-year survival of patients who have metastatic disease is now reported to be approximately

70%.[9,70,71] By contrast, before the introduction of imatinib, the median survival after surgical resection of recurrent GIST was only 15 months.[70]

Because imatinib rarely induces a complete response, and median time to progression with imatinib therapy is less than 24 months, a multimodal approach using surgical resection in conjunction with imatinib therapy to treat recurrent metastatic GIST is highly desirable. In a recent study from the authors' institution,[58] 40 patients who had metastatic GIST were treated with tyrosine kinase inhibitors for a median of 15 months before surgical resection. After surgery, 20 patients who had responsive disease based on preoperative serial radiologic imaging had a 2-year progression-free survival of 61% and 2-year overall survival of 100% (**Fig. 6**). In contrast, 13 patients who experienced focal resistance of their disease progressed at a median of 12 months postoperatively, with a 2-year overall survival of 36%. There were seven patients who had multifocal resistant disease, and they progressed postoperatively at a median of 3 months and experienced a 1-year overall survival of 36%. Based on these results, selected patients with metastatic GIST who have responsive disease or focal resistance to imatinib may benefit from resection. In contrast, in patients who have metastatic GIST and multifocal resistance, surgery generally is not indicated.[58] Similar results were observed by Gronchi and colleagues[72] in a study employing 38 patients with advanced GIST who underwent surgery following a variable period of imatinib therapy. Additionally, Raut and colleagues[73] published their series of 69 patients with advanced GIST who underwent surgery and concluded that patients with advanced GIST exhibiting stable disease or minimal progression on kinase inhibitor therapy have prolonged overall survival after debulking procedures. Surgery has little to offer in patients who have generalized progression of disease while on therapy.

The authors propose that the risk of developing imatinib resistance is proportional to the amount of residual viable GIST. Therefore, once maximal response to imatinib occurs (generally after 2 to 6 months of therapy), the authors evaluate patients for complete resection. Imatinib therapy is continued postoperatively to delay or prevent subsequent disease recurrence, although the optional duration of therapy is unknown.[31] A recent study showed an increase in the rate of progressive disease when imatinib was interrupted.[74]

The success of imatinib in treating patients who have GIST is defined by lack of disease progression, rather than shrinkage of existing tumors.[75] When metabolic imaging and anatomic imaging are combined, GISTs that respond to molecular therapy may be stable in size but demonstrate areas of necrosis. When using these criteria, 12% of patients with GIST who are treated with imatinib demonstrate primary resistance, defined as progression within the first 6 months of imatinib treatment.[75] Clinical studies have demonstrated that the location of mutations in the pathogenic kinase is an important factor in treatment response and development of resistance to imatinib.[76] Patients who experience primary resistance usually express both wild-type KIT and PDGFRα, or contain mutations in exon 9 of KIT or a PDGFRα with a D842 V mutation.[43,77]

Secondary or late resistance therefore occurs in patients who initially have demonstrated stabilization of their disease for at least 6 months. Unfortunately, most patients who initially demonstrate a clinical response to imatinib subsequently will develop (secondary) resistance, as a result of selection for additional point mutations in the KIT kinase domains.[78] Usually, most resistant GISTs with secondary mutation have primary mutations in exon 11. The second site mutations are mainly substitutions involving exons 13, 14, and 17 of KIT, corresponding to the kinase domain. Recent studies suggest that patients with primary KIT mutations in exon 13 K642E and in exon 14 T670I have acquired resistance to imatinib.[78]

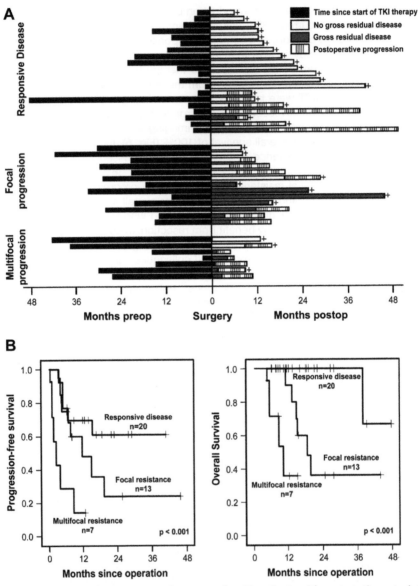

Fig. 6. (A) Timeline of treatment and outcome for 40 patients with metastatic gastrointestinal stromal tumor (GIST) treated with molecular therapy and then surgery. Each patient is represented by a horizontal bar. The patients are grouped by their response at the time of surgery to tyrosine kinase inhibitor (TKI) therapy. The time period from the start of TKI therapy to surgery is shown by the black boxes. All patients were operated upon at time zero. After surgery, patients had either no gross residual disease (*white boxes*) or gross residual disease (*gray boxes*). Postoperative progression is shown by the striped boxes. A plus sign designates the patients who were alive at last follow-up; the other patients have died of disease. (B) Progression-free and overall survival after resection of metastatic GIST. (*From* DeMatteo RP, Ronald P, Maki RG, et al. Results of tyrosine kinase inhibitor therapy followed by surgical resection for metastatic gastrointestinal stromal tumor. Ann Surg 2007;245:347; with permission.)

There is general agreement that multifocal resistance to imatinib should be treated with another targeted agent such as sunitinib, which has activity against KIT and PDGFRα, and the vascular endothelial cell growth factor (VEGF) and fms-related tyrosine kinase 3 (Flt3) receptors. Sunitinib also may have activity in GIST harboring secondary KIT mutations.[79] In 48 patients who were treated with sunitinib after disease progression with imatinib therapy, there were 20 patients with stable disease and 6 who achieved a partial response. Increasing the imatinib dose from 400 to 800 mg/d may overcome or balance the effects of drug resistance to imatinib and increase progression-free time. The success of this strategy appears to be limited, however, except in tumors with primary mutations in KIT exon 9. For other GISTs, the dose of imatinib required to overcome drug resistance or delay progression is prohibitively high. Several other agents are in clinical trials, as different agents interact with alternate moieties on the KIT protein, and resistance to one agent may not preclude a therapeutic benefit from another. Further understanding of the mechanisms of resistance to imatinib may allow for the delay or prevention of this phenomenon, in addition to using additional targeted therapies.[78] A proposed algorithm for treatment of primary and recurrent metastatic GIST is outlined (**Fig. 7**), and has been revised as the awaited results of phase 2 and 3 ACOSOG trials are now out, and phase 2 RTOG trial finings will be published in the near future.

SUMMARY

Imatinib treatment for GIST has become paradigm of oncogene treatment of solid tumors. As a consequence, the treatment of GIST has evolved rapidly, with dramatic changes in clinical practice. Nevertheless, time has shown the limitations of treating GIST with this single agent alone, as resistance to tyrosine kinase inhibitors is an emerging clinical dilemma. Surgical resection still remains the only chance for cure. However, recent studies have begun to delineate effective ways to integrate surgery and targeted therapy or reduce recurrence after resection of primary disease and to prolong survival in metastatic disease. The lessons learned in GIST, along with ongoing and future investigations, will be extremely relevant to the potential use of molecular therapy for other cancers.

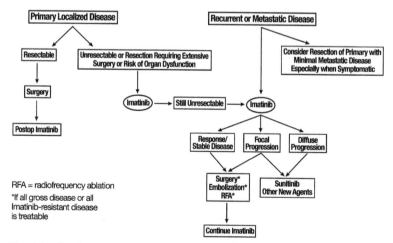

Fig. 7. Algorithm for the treatment of gastrointestinal stromal tumor. (*From* Gold JS, DeMatteo RP. Combined surgical and molecular therapy: the gastrointestinal stromal tumor model. Ann Surg 2006;244:176; with permission.)

REFERENCES

1. Mazur MT, Clark HB. Gastric stromal tumors. Reappraisal of histogenesis. Am J Surg Pathol 1983;7(6):507–19.
2. Howe JR, Karnell LH, Scott-Conner C. Small bowel sarcoma: analysis of survival from the National Cancer Data Base. Ann Surg Oncol 2001;8(6):496–508.
3. Hirota S, Isozaki K, Moriyama Y, et al. Gain-of-function mutations of c-kit in human gastrointestinal stromal tumors. Science 1998;279(5350):577–80.
4. Suster S. Gastrointestinal stromal tumors. Semin Diagn Pathol 1996;13(4):297–313.
5. Rubin BP, Singer S, Tsao C, et al. KIT activation is a ubiquitous feature of gastrointestinal stromal tumors. Cancer Res 2001;61(22):8118–21.
6. Antonescu CR, Sommer G, Sarran L, et al. Association of KIT exon 9 mutations with nongastric primary site and aggressive behavior: KIT mutation analysis and clinical correlates of 120 gastrointestinal stromal tumors. Clin Cancer Res 2003;9(9):3329–37.
7. Heinrich MC, Corless CL, Duensing A, et al. PDGFRA activating mutations in gastrointestinal stromal tumors. Science 2003;299(5607):708–10.
8. Joensuu H, Roberts PJ, Sarlomo-Rikala M, et al. Effect of the tyrosine kinase inhibitor STI571 in a patient with a metastatic gastrointestinal stromal tumor. N Engl J Med 2001;344(14):1052–6.
9. Demetri GD, von Mehren M, Blanke CD, et al. Efficacy and safety of imatinib mesylate in advanced gastrointestinal stromal tumors. N Engl J Med 2002;347(7):472–80.
10. DeMatteo RP, Lewis JJ, Leung D, et al. Two hundred gastrointestinal stromal tumors: recurrence patterns and prognostic factors for survival. Ann Surg 2000;231(1):51–8.
11. Thomas RM, Sobin LH. Gastrointestinal cancer. Cancer 1995;75(1 Suppl):154–70.
12. Demetri GD, Baker LH, Benjamin RS, et al. Soft tissue sarcoma. J Natl Compr Canc Netw 2007;5(4):364–99.
13. Demetri GD, Benjamin RS, Blanke CD, et al. NCCN Task Force report: management of patients with gastrointestinal stromal tumor (GIST)—update of the NCCN clinical practice guidelines. J Natl Compr Canc Netw 2007;5(Suppl 2):S1–29 [quiz S30].
14. Nilsson B, Bumming P, Meis-Kindblom JM, et al. Gastrointestinal stromal tumors: the incidence, prevalence, clinical course, and prognostication in the preimatinib mesylate era—a population-based study in western Sweden. Cancer 2005;103(4):821–9.
15. Nishida T, Hirota S, Taniguchi M, et al. Familial gastrointestinal stromal tumours with germline mutation of the KIT gene. Nat Genet 1998;19(4):323–4.
16. Chompret A, Kannengiesser C, Barrois M, et al. PDGFRA germline mutation in a family with multiple cases of gastrointestinal stromal tumor. Gastroenterology 2004;126(1):318–21.
17. Takazawa Y, Sakurai S, Sakuma Y, et al. Gastrointestinal stromal tumors of neurofibromatosis type I (von Recklinghausen's disease). Am J Surg Pathol 2005;29(6):755–63.
18. Carney JA. The triad of gastric epithelioid leiomyosarcoma, functioning extraadrenal paraganglioma, and pulmonary chondroma. Cancer 1979;43(1):374–82.
19. Emory TS, Sobin LH, Lukes L, et al. Prognosis of gastrointestinal smooth-muscle (stromal) tumors: dependence on anatomic site. Am J Surg Pathol 1999;23(1):82–7.

20. Graadt van Roggen JF, van Velthuysen ML, Hogendoorn PC. The histopatholog-ical differential diagnosis of gastrointestinal stromal tumours. J Clin Pathol 2001; 54(2):96–102.
21. Miettinen M, Sarlomo-Rikala M, Sobin LH, et al. Esophageal stromal tumors: a clin-icopathologic, immunohistochemical, and molecular genetic study of 17 cases and comparison with esophageal leiomyomas and leiomyosarcomas. Am J Surg Pathol 2000;24(2):211–22.
22. Agaram NP, Laquaglia MP, Ustun B, et al. Molecular characterization of pediatric gastrointestinal stromal tumors. Clin Cancer Res 2008;14(10):3204–15.
23. Ueyama T, Guo KJ, Hashimoto H, et al. A clinicopathologic and immunohisto-chemical study of gastrointestinal stromal tumors. Cancer 1992;69(4):947–55.
24. Hurlimann J, Gardiol D. Gastrointestinal stromal tumours: an immunohistochem-ical study of 165 cases. Histopathology 1991;19(4):311–20.
25. Yagihashi S, Kimura M, Kurotaki H, et al. Gastric submucosal tumours of neuro-genic origin with neuroaxonal and Schwann cell elements. J Pathol 1987;153(1): 41–50.
26. Kindblom LG, Remotti HE, Aldenborg F, et al. Gastrointestinal pacemaker cell tumor (GIPACT): gastrointestinal stromal tumors show phenotypic characteristics of the interstitial cells of Cajal. Am J Pathol 1998;152(5):1259–69.
27. Bickenbach K, Wilcox R, Veerapong J, et al. A review of resistance patterns and phenotypic changes in gastrointestinal stromal tumors following imatinib mesy-late therapy. J Gastrointest Surg 2007;11(6):758–66.
28. Antonescu CR, Busam KJ, Francone TD, et al. L576P KIT mutation in anal mela-nomas correlates with KIT protein expression and is sensitive to specific kinase inhibition. Int J Cancer 2007;121(2):257–64.
29. Fletcher CD, Berman JJ, Corless C, et al. Diagnosis of gastrointestinal stromal tumors: a consensus approach. Hum Pathol 2002;33(5):459–65.
30. Katz SC, DeMatteo RP. Gastrointestinal stromal tumors and leiomyosarcomas. J Surg Oncol 2008;97(4):350–9.
31. van der Zwan SM, DeMatteo RP. Gastrointestinal stromal tumor: 5 years later. Cancer 2005;104(9):1781–8.
32. Medeiros F, Corless CL, Duensing A, et al. KIT-negative gastrointestinal stromal tumors: proof of concept and therapeutic implications. Am J Surg Pathol 2004; 28(7):889–94.
33. Tzen CY, Mau BL. Analysis of CD117-negative gastrointestinal stromal tumors. World J Gastroenterol 2005;11(7):1052–5.
34. Dematteo RP, Gold JS, Saran L, et al. Tumor mitotic rate, size, and location inde-pendently predict recurrence after resection of primary gastrointestinal stromal tumor (GIST). Cancer 2008;112(3):608–15.
35. Franquemont DW. Differentiation and risk assessment of gastrointestinal stromal tumors. Am J Clin Pathol 1995;103(1):41–7.
36. Ranchod M, Kempson RL. Smooth muscle tumors of the gastrointestinal tract and retroperitoneum: a pathologic analysis of 100 cases. Cancer 1977;39(1):255–62.
37. Sommer G, Agosti V, Ehlers I, et al. Gastrointestinal stromal tumors in a mouse model by targeted mutation of the KIT receptor tyrosine kinase. Proc Natl Acad Sci U S A 2003;100(11):6706–11.
38. Tsujimura T, Morimoto M, Hashimoto K, et al. Constitutive activation of c-kit in FMA3 murine mastocytoma cells caused by deletion of seven amino acids at the juxtamembrane domain. Blood 1996;87(1):273–83.
39. Tian Q, Frierson HF Jr, Krystal GW, et al. Activating c-kit gene mutations in human germ cell tumors. Am J Pathol 1999;154(6):1643–7.

40. Kanakura Y, Ikeda H, Kitayama H, et al. Expression, function, and activation of the proto-oncogene c-kit product in human leukemia cells. Leuk Lymphoma 1993; 10(1–2):35–41.
41. Cohen PS, Chan JP, Lipkunskaya M, et al. Expression of stem cell factor and c-kit in human neuroblastoma. The Children's Cancer Group. Blood 1994;84(10): 3465–72.
42. Lux ML, Rubin BP, Biase TL, et al. KIT extracellular and kinase domain mutations in gastrointestinal stromal tumors. Am J Pathol 2000;156(3):791–5.
43. Joensuu H. Gastrointestinal stromal tumor (GIST). Ann Oncol 2006;17(Suppl 10): x280–6.
44. Breiner JA, Meis-Kindblom J, Kindblom LG, et al. Loss of 14q and 22q in gastro-intestinal stromal tumors (pacemaker cell tumors). Cancer Genet Cytogenet 2000;120(2):111–6.
45. Gold JS, Dematteo RP. Combined surgical and molecular therapy: the gastroin-testinal stromal tumor model. Ann Surg 2006;244(2):176–84.
46. Dematteo RP, Maki RG, Antonescu C, et al. Targeted molecular therapy for cancer: the application of STI571 to gastrointestinal stromal tumor. Curr Probl Surg 2003;40(3):144–93.
47. Miettinen M, El-Rifai W, HL Sobin L, et al. Evaluation of malignancy and prognosis of gastrointestinal stromal tumors: a review. Hum Pathol 2002;33(5):478–83.
48. Shiu MH, Farr GH, Papachristou DN, et al. Myosarcomas of the stomach: natural history, prognostic factors, and management. Cancer 1982;49(1):177–87.
49. Ng EH, Pollock RE, Munsell MF, et al. Prognostic factors influencing survival in gastrointestinal leiomyosarcomas. Implications for surgical management and staging. Ann Surg 1992;215(1):68–77.
50. Rudolph P, Gloeckner K, Parwaresch R, et al. Immunophenotype, proliferation, DNA ploidy, and biological behavior of gastrointestinal stromal tumors: a multivar-iate clinicopathologic study. Hum Pathol 1998;29(8):791–800.
51. Goldblum JR, Appelman HD. Stromal tumors of the duodenum. A histologic and immunohistochemical study of 20 cases. Am J Surg Pathol 1995;19(1):71–80.
52. Kiyabu MT, Bishop PC, Parker JW, et al. Smooth muscle tumors of the gastrointestinal tract. Flow cytometric quantitation of DNA and nuclear antigen content and correlation with histologic grade. Am J Surg Pathol 1988;12(12): 954–60.
53. Cooper PN, Quirke P, Hardy GJ, et al. A flow cytometric, clinical, and histological study of stromal neoplasms of the gastrointestinal tract. Am J Surg Pathol 1992; 16(2):163–70.
54. Gunther T, Schneider-Stock R, Hackel C, et al. Telomerase activity and expres-sion of hTRT and hTR in gastrointestinal stromal tumors in comparison with extra-gastrointestinal sarcomas. Clin Cancer Res 2000;6(5):1811–8.
55. Prenen H, Deroose C, Vermaelen P, et al. Establishment of a mouse gastrointes-tinal stromal tumour model and evaluation of response to imatinib by small animal positron emission tomography. Anticancer Res 2006;26(2A):1247–52.
56. Tran T, Davila JA, El-Serag HB. The epidemiology of malignant gastrointestinal stromal tumors: an analysis of 1458 cases from 1992 to 2000. Am J Gastroenterol 2005;100(1):162–8.
57. Ng EH, Pollock RE, Romsdahl MM. Prognostic implications of patterns of failure for gastrointestinal leiomyosarcomas. Cancer 1992;69(6):1334–41.
58. DeMatteo R, Ronald P, Maki RG, et al. Results of tyrosine kinase inhibitor therapy followed by surgical resection for metastatic gastrointestinal stromal tumor. Ann Surg 2007;245:347–52.

59. DeMatteo RP. The GIST of targeted cancer therapy: a tumor (gastrointestinal stromal tumor), a mutated gene (c-kit), and a molecular inhibitor (STI571). Ann Surg Oncol 2002;9(9):831–9.
60. Edmonson JH. Chemotherapeutic approaches to soft tissue sarcomas. Semin Surg Oncol 1994;10(5):357–63.
61. Edmonson JH, Ryan LM, Blum RH, et al. Randomized comparison of doxorubicin alone versus ifosfamide plus doxorubicin or mitomycin, doxorubicin, and cisplatin against advanced soft tissue sarcomas. J Clin Oncol 1993;11(7):1269–75.
62. Demetri GD. ET-743: the US experience in sarcomas of soft tissues. Anticancer Drugs 2002;13(Suppl 1):S7–9.
63. DeMatteo RP, Shah A, Fong Y, et al. Results of hepatic resection for sarcoma metastatic to liver. Ann Surg 2001;234(4):540–7 [discussion: 547–8].
64. D'Amato G, Steinert DM, McAuliffe JC, et al. Update on the biology and therapy of gastrointestinal stromal tumors. Cancer Control 2005;12(1):44–56.
65. Savage DG, Antman KH. Imatinib mesylate–a new oral targeted therapy. N Engl J Med 2002;346(9):683–93.
66. Druker BJ, Talpaz M, Resta DJ, et al. Efficacy and safety of a specific inhibitor of the BCR-ABL tyrosine kinase in chronic myeloid leukemia. N Engl J Med 2001; 344(14):1031–7.
67. DeMatteo RP, Owzar, K, Antonescu, CR, et al. Efficacy of adjuvant imatinib mesylate following complete resection of localized, primary gastrointestinal stromal tumor (GIST) at high risk of recurrence: The U.S. Intergroup phase II trial ACOSOG Z9000. 2008 Paper presented at the Gastrointestinal Cancers Symposium, January 25–27, 2008, Orlando, FL.
68. Dematteo R. Adjuvant imatinib mesylate in patients with primary high risk gastrointestinal stromal tumor (GIST) following complete resection: Safety results from the U.S. Intergroup Phase II trial ACOSOG Z9000. Presented at ASCO, May 13–17, 2005, Orlando, FL.
69. DeMatteo RP, Owzar K, Maki R, et al. Adjuvant imatinib mesylate increases recurrence free survival (RFS) in patients with completely resected localized primary gastrointestinal stromal tumor (GIST): North American Intergroup Phase III trial ACOSOG Z9001. Presented at the 2007 ASCO Annual Meeting, June 1–5, 2007, Chicago, IL.
70. Verweij J, Casali PG, Zalcberg J, et al. Progression-free survival in gastrointestinal stromal tumours with high-dose imatinib: randomised trial. Lancet 2004; 364(9440):1127–34.
71. van Oosterom AT, Judson I, Verweij J, et al. Safety and efficacy of imatinib (STI571) in metastatic gastrointestinal stromal tumours: a phase I study. Lancet 2001;358(9291):1421–3.
72. Gronchi A, Fiore M, Miselli F, et al. Surgery of residual disease following molecular-targeted therapy with imatinib mesylate in advanced/metastatic GIST. Ann Surg 2007;245(3):341–6.
73. Raut CP, Posner M, Desai J, et al. Surgical management of advanced gastrointestinal stromal tumors after treatment with targeted systemic therapy using kinase inhibitors. J Clin Oncol 2006;24(15):2325–31.
74. La Cense A, Perol D, Ray-Coquard I. Interruption of imatinib (IM) in GIST patients with advanced disease: updated results of the prospective French Sarcoma Group randomized phase III trial on survival and quality of life. J Clin Oncol 2005;23(16S):9031.
75. Van Glabbeke M, Verweij J, Casali PG, et al. Initial and late resistance to imatinib in advanced gastrointestinal stromal tumors are predicted by different prognostic

factors: a European Organisation for Research and Treatment of Cancer-Italian Sarcoma Group-Australasian Gastrointestinal Trials Group study. J Clin Oncol 2005;23(24):5795–804.

76. Judson I, Demetri G. Advances in the treatment of gastrointestinal stromal tumours. Ann Oncol 2007;18(Suppl 10):x20–4.

77. Heinrich MC, Corless CL, Demetri GD, et al. Kinase mutations and imatinib response in patients with metastatic gastrointestinal stromal tumor. J Clin Oncol 2003;21(23):4342–9.

78. Antonescu CR, Besmer P, Guo T, et al. Acquired resistance to imatinib in gastro-intestinal stromal tumor occurs through secondary gene mutation. Clin Cancer Res 2005;11(11):4182–90.

79. Prenen H, Cools J, Mentens N, et al. Efficacy of the kinase inhibitor SU11248 against gastrointestinal stromal tumor mutants refractory to imatinib mesylate. Clin Cancer Res 2006;12(8):2622–7.

Cardiovascular Effects of Tyrosine Kinase Inhibitors Used for Gastrointestinal Stromal Tumors

Vishnu Chintalgattu, PhD[a], Shalin S. Patel[a], Aarif Y. Khakoo, MD[b],*

KEYWORDS
- Gastrointestinal stromal tumor • Cancer • Cardiotoxicity
- Tyrosine kinase inhibitors • Imatinib • Sunitinib

CARDIOTOXICITY ATTRIBUTABLE TO ANTHRACYCLINES IN PATIENTS WHO HAVE GASTROINTESTINAL STROMAL TUMORS

Of the traditional chemotherapeutic agents used in the treatment of sarcomas, the anthracyclines are most strongly associated with cardiotoxicity. Cardiac dysfunction attributable to anthracycline-based chemotherapy in patients who have sarcoma has been well recognized since the 1970s.[1] There is a clear dose dependence in the cardiotoxicity of anthracyclines. Early studies reported the incidence of heart failure attributable to anthracycline-based chemotherapy to be 4% when the total cumulative dosage is less than 550 mg/m^2, ranging to as high as 30% when the cumulative dosage is greater than 600 mg/m^2.[2] Measures to limit cardiotoxicity attributable to anthracycline-based chemotherapies, such as use of regimens that limit the total cumulative dosage of drug, employment of methods to monitor cardiac function carefully during treatment,[3] and use of a liposomal-based formulation of doxorubicin,[4] seem to have reduced the incidence of this devastating complication. Cardiotoxicity attributable to anthracyclines remains a major complication of this well-established sarcoma therapy, however, as evidenced by the fact that patients who have

Data presented in this review were obtained by searching the PubMed database. The key words used for searches were cardiotoxicity, chemotherapy, TKI, GIST, imatinib, sunitinib, and dasatinib.

[a] Department of Cardiology, University of Texas, M.D. Anderson Cancer Center, Institute of Biosciences and Technology, Room 718, 2121 West Holcombe Boulevard, Houston, TX 77030, USA

[b] Department of Cardiology, University of Texas, M.D. Anderson Cancer Center, 1515 Holcombe Boulevard, Houston, TX 77030, USA

* Corresponding author.

E-mail address: aykhakoo@mdanderson.org (A.Y. Khakoo).

cardiomyopathy attributable to anthracyclines are among the groups with the worst prognosis when compared with groups of patients who have other forms of cardiomyopathy, including ischemic heart disease.[5] In fact, adult survivors of childhood cancers who received traditional cancer therapy, including anthracyclines, are at an even higher risk for cardiovascular disease than of recurrent malignancy.[6,7] Dose-limiting cardiovascular complications of chemotherapeutic agents, such as the anthracyclines, coupled with a quest for more efficacious cancer therapies and an increased understanding of the molecular biology of cancer have served to drive the development of molecularly targeted cancer therapy.

THE PROMISE OF MOLECULARLY TARGETED THERAPY

The advent of small tyrosine kinase inhibitors (TKIs) revolutionized the treatment of cancers, including chronic myeloid leukemia (CML), renal cell carcinoma (RCC), and colon carcinoma, and has also changed the therapeutic landscape for patients who have gastrointestinal stromal tumors (GISTs).[8-12] These target-based cancer drugs are tailored to the genetic mutations of each cancer. The use of imatinib as a therapy targeting the Abl kinase, the essential dysregulated signaling molecule in patients who have CML, represents a new paradigm in rational drug design and has shown remarkable efficacy in the treatment of patients who have early-chronic-phase and advanced-stage CML.[13,14] Based on increased survival rates of patients treated with imatinib, there has been a new shift in the paradigm of cancer prognosis. Cancers that previously were fatal and incurable are now looked at as manageable chronic diseases, if not curable ailments.[15]

The promise of molecularly targeted cancer therapy is based on the premise that by specifically inhibiting molecules associated with tumor growth, such therapies should be highly effective in treating cancer without adversely affecting normal organs,[16] in contrast to traditional chemotherapeutic agents, such as anthracyclines, which are effective in the treatment of several malignancies yet can result in a cancer survivor who has devastating cardiac disease. As more individuals survive their cancer, the development of new therapies that are effective and have minimal long-term adverse cardiac effects is of the utmost importance.

Although targeted cancer therapies are typically aimed at molecules that are overexpressed in cancer cells, the fact remains that many receptor tyrosine kinases (TKs) are expressed in normal tissues, and these molecules may play a role in normal physiology of many organ systems, including the cardiovascular system. A striking example of this was seen in the treatment of patients who have breast cancer with the monoclonal antibody trastuzumab, whose target is the product of the Her 2/Neu gene, the receptor TK ErbB2. Her2/Neu overexpression is a critical factor in the progression of several forms of breast cancer.[17] Seven percent of patients treated with trastuzumab as a second-line agent after anthracycline treatment develop cardiomyopathy, and 29% of patients treated concurrently with trastuzumab and anthracyclines develop cardiomyopathy.[18] Subsequent work by molecular cardiologists led to elucidation of a critical role for ErbB2 in cardiac development and in the cardiac response to physiologic stress.[19,20]

Targeted anticancer agents that are specific to dysregulated TKs in malignant cells are divided into two general classes: monoclonal antibodies, which specifically target extracellular receptors, and small-molecule TKIs. During the development of TKIs, it was thought that TKs were relatively quiescent at physiologic levels in comparison to constitutively active TKs in cancers. Therefore, it was thought that TKIs treat the cancers specifically with minimal or no cardiotoxic effects.[15] Preclinical and clinical observations have revealed that subsets of TKIs in clinical use today are potentially cardiotoxic, however (**Table 1**).[21–24] In this review, the authors describe what is known clinically and preclinically about the effects of small-molecule TKIs that are currently used in the treatment of GISTs.

IMATINIB MESYLATE

Imatinib mesylate (Gleevec; Novartis, East Hanover, New Jersey) is an ATP-competitive small-molecule TKI whose principal cancer molecular targets are Abl kinase for CML and c-kit and platelet-derived growth factor receptor (PDGFR)-α for GISTs. Imatinib also inhibits the TKs PDGFRβ, ABL-related gene, and FMS-like tyrosine kinase receptor-3(Flt3). As a result of the clinical efficacy of imatinib during clinical trials, it was approved by the US Food and Drug Administration (FDA) for the treatment of Philadelphia chromosome-positive CML (based on its effects on Abl), gastrointestinal stromal tumor (based on its effect on c-kit or PDGFRα), acute lymphatic leukemia (ALL), and chronic myelomonocytic or eosinophilic leukemia (based on its effects on PDGFR).[25] In pH+ ALL and CML, imatinib therapy substantially increased the rate of remission and increased survival in refractory and newly diagnosed patients.[26,27] In addition, imatinib may have several other potential therapeutic indications, such as in the treatment of pulmonary hypertension,[28] use as a cholesterol-lowering agent,[29] and, as recently demonstrated, in the treatment of ischemic stroke.[30]

Until recently, imatinib was hailed for its impressive targeted anticancer therapeutic effects and minimal side-effect profile, especially when compared with toxicities seen attributable to traditional chemotherapy.[31] Concern for cardiotoxicity attributable to imatinib was first raised based on a study by Kerkela and colleagues,[22] however, who documented cardiomyopathy in mice treated with imatinib at clinically relevant dosages and demonstrated that imatinib treatment causes a significant loss of left ventricular (LV) mass and a decline in LV function. To explain the effects of imatinib on murine cardiac function, Kerkela and colleagues[22] showed that hearts from

Table 1
Cardiotoxic effects of tyrosine kinase inhibitors used to treat gastrointestinal stromal tumors

Agents	Targets	Cardiovascular Toxicity
Agents currently used to treat GISTs		
Imatinib	KIT, PDGFRα/β, Abl, Flt-3, LCK	HF
Sunitinib	KIT, PDGFRα/β, VEGFR1-3, RET, CSF-1R	HF, HTN
Agents Under Clinical Investigation		
Vatalanib	KIT, PDGFRα/β, VEGFR1-3	Unknown
Nilotinib	KIT, PDGFRα/β, Abl	QT prolongation, sudden death
Masatinib	KIT, PDGFRα/β, FGFR3	Unknown
Sorafenib	KIT, PDGFRβ, VEGFR-2/3, Raf, Flt-3, RET	HF, HTN
AMG706	KIT, PDGFRα/β, VEGFR1-3, RET	Unknown
PKC412	KIT, PDGFRα/β, VEGFR2	Unknown
AZD2171	KIT, PDGFRα/β, VEGFR1-3, Flt-3	Unknown

Abbreviations: Abl, Abl oncogene; CSF-1R, colony stimulating factor-1 receptor; FGFR3, fibroblast growth factor receptor-3; Flt-3, fms-like tyrosine kinase receptor-3; HF, heart failure; HTN, hypertension; KIT, stem cell factor receptor; LCK, lymphocyte-specific protein tyrosine kinase; PDGFR, platelet-derived growth factor receptor; RET, RET proto-oncogene; VEGFR1-3, vascular endothelial growth factor receptor; FGFR3, fibroblast growth factor receptor-3.

imatinib-treated mice displayed morphologic mitochondrial abnormalities. Furthermore, cultured cardiac myocytes treated with imatinib displayed mitochondrial toxicity, depletion of ATP, and activation of the endoplasmic reticulum (ER) stress response, a cellular protective mechanism that is activated after several physiologic conditions associated with energy depletion. Kerkela and colleagues[22] identified a subset of imatinib-treated patients without a history of heart disease who developed heart failure after treatment with imatinib. Strikingly, endomyocardial biopsies from these patients revealed mitochondrial abnormalities similar to those observed in imatinib-treated mice, further emphasizing the importance of the preclinical findings.

Mechanistically, Kerkela and colleagues[22] linked the effects of imatinib on the heart to inhibition of Abl kinase, whose role in cardiac function was previously not well established. Introducing a genetically modified form of Abl kinase that was resistant to the effects of imatinib into cardiomyocytes partially rescued them from imatinib-induced mitochondrial dysfunction. Work by Fernandez and colleagues[32] further supported the contention that the cardiotoxicity of imatinib in the mouse was at least partially attributable to the effects of imatinib on cardiac Abl kinase. Importantly, Fernandez and colleagues[22] were able to replicate the effects of imatinib on cardiac function reported by Kerkela and colleagues.[22] In addition, Fernandez and colleagues[32] designed a structurally re-engineered form of imatinib (known as WBZ4) that does not inhibit Abl but retains its inhibitory activity of stem cell factor receptor (KIT). In vivo, this correlated with retained antitumor activity in a murine KIT-dependent GIST model. When compared with imatinib, however, WBZ4 had decreased adverse effects on cardiac mitochondrial function and cardiac contractility.

Although the study by Kerkela and colleagues[22] only reported congestive heart failure in 10 imatinib-treated patients and did not report the actual incidence of imatinib-associated heart failure, their report led to great concerns about the cardiac safety of imatinib, by health care providers and among the general public,[33] and ultimately led the drug manufacturer to revise its drug labeling to include warnings regarding possible congestive heart failure. Several letters[34–36] in response to the publication by Kerkela and colleagues[37] reported a low incidence of clinically significant heart failure associated with imatinib in clinical trial settings, although none of these letters referenced studies in which routine prospective monitoring of cardiac function was performed. Subsequent reports of retrospective analyses of adverse events in patients who had GISTs[38] and in patients who had CML[39] presented data reporting an incidence of heart failure in imatinib-treated patients of 1% to 2%. In the CML study,[39] the investigators used an age-matched cohort to argue that there was no excess in the incidence of cardiotoxicity in imatinib-treated patients compared with what one would expect in the treated population without exposure to imatinib. These conclusions, however, must be viewed with some caution in light of the fact that none were based on studies with programs designed to monitor cardiac function explicitly, and assessment of cardiac events was based primarily on adverse event reports, which may significantly underestimate the incidence of cardiac disease in a cancer population. Establishing the diagnosis of heart failure based on history and physical examination alone is notoriously challenging,[15] and in patients who have cancer, who often have symptoms attributable to their cancer that can overlap with the cardinal symptoms of congestive heart failure, clinical diagnosis is even more challenging. Furthermore, lower extremity edema, a common adverse effect of imatinib therapy, can mask edema caused by congestive heart failure in these patients.

Notably, a recent study in patients who had GISTs treated with imatinib used prospective monitoring with serum levels of B-type natriuretic peptide (BNP) to determine the incidence of heart failure associated with imatinib in patients who had

GISTs.[40] In this small study (55 patients) with short-term follow-up of 3 months, 2 patients experienced substantial increases in BNP levels over a 3-month follow-up period, suggesting an incidence of heart failure associated with imatinib therapy in the range of 4% in patients who have GISTs.

The preclinical findings showing cardiotoxicity in mouse models warrant further, well-designed, prospective studies with objective cardiac monitoring to determine the incidence and clinical significance of heart failure attributable to imatinib in patients who have GISTs. While we await such studies, the wealth of currently available studies, most of which are in patients who have CML, suggest that cardiac complications attributable to imatinib are manageable and should not be a reason to withhold imatinib therapy from patients who have cancer and would derive benefit.

SUNTINIB MALATE

Several small-molecule inhibitors of multiple receptor TKs have been approved in the treatment of a variety of malignancies, and many more are in various stages of development. Although the broader biologic activity of these molecules may contribute to a greater therapeutic effect, there is concern that off-target toxicities, including effects on the cardiovascular system, may be an unintended consequence of this enhanced biologic activity.[41] Sunitinib malate (SU11248, Sutent; Pfizer, Inc., New York, New York) is a multitargeted TKI with profound antiangiogenic activity. Sunitinib's potency as an antitumor agent arises from its inhibition of multiple molecular targets, such as KIT, PDGFRα/β, vascular endothelial growth factor receptor (VEGFR1) -3, RET proto-oncogene (RET), and colony-stimulating factor-1 receptor, many of which are prominent TKs that are mutated or overexpressed in RCC and GIST. Sunitinib has been approved by the FDA for the treatment of patients who have advanced RCC and for patients who have imatinib-resistant GISTs. Questions about the cardiac safety of sunitinib emerged from early clinical trials of the drug. In an early study of patients who had GISTs, 10% of sunitinib-treated patients experienced left ventricular dysfunction (LVD) compared with 3% treated with placebo.[42] Similarly, patients who had metastatic RCC treated with sunitinib developed LVD 15% of the time.[43] Additionally, 4.6% of patients treated with sunitinib monotherapy for RCC have been reported to have LVD, as defined by a reduction in LV ejection fraction greater than 20%.[44] Recently, clinical reports with more detailed descriptions of heart failure associated with sunitinib malate suggest that cardiac dysfunction associated with sunitinib therapy is a clinically important adverse effect with significant morbidity and mortality. In sunitinib-treated patients who had GISTs, Chu and colleagues[21] reported a 28% incidence of an absolute reduction in cardiac ejection fraction of 10% or greater, along with an 8% incidence of congestive heart failure over a follow-up period of 33 weeks. Notably, Chu and colleagues[21] found a parallel dose-dependent increase in blood pressure with sunitinib therapy, suggesting a mechanistic link between hypertension and heart failure in these patients. Consistent with these findings, the authors reported heart failure in sunitinib-treated patients associated with significant morbidity and mortality. In the authors' study,[23] a referral-based study of patients treated with sunitinib at M.D. Anderson Cancer Center over a 1-year period, they found that 3% of treated patients developed congestive heart failure and LVD. The authors found that cardiac dysfunction associated with sunitinib therapy improves after cessation of the drug in some but not all patients who develop cardiac dysfunction. The referral-based nature of that study suggests that the incidence of heart failure associated with sunitinib treatment is likely greater than what the authors reported. Similar to the findings of Chu and colleagues,[21] the authors found that sunitinib-treated patients who developed heart failure had marked increases in systolic and diastolic blood pressure. Furthermore, heart failure associated with sunitinib therapy occurred soon after initiation of drug (mean onset of 29 days after treatment initiation), suggesting to the authors that acute increases in blood pressure, coupled with a toxic effect of sunitinib on cardiomyocytes, may impair the ability of the heart to respond to these increases in blood pressure, resulting in heart failure in subsets of treated patients. In support of this mechanistic hypothesis, Chu and colleagues[21] found that sunitinib caused direct mitochondrial toxicity to cultured cardiac myocytes, which would be predicted to impair the cardiomyocyte stress response.

FUTURE CONSIDERATIONS

As we begin to understand possible additional cardiotoxicities attributable to TKIs used for the treatment of GISTs, there are several critical questions that are still not well understood. First and foremost, prospective studies of potentially cardiotoxic TKIs, such as imatinib and sunitinib, that include prospective assessment of cardiac function and long-term follow-up are needed to define the true incidence of adverse cardiac events, such as hypertension, cardiac dysfunction, cardiac ischemia, and congestive heart failure. Such studies should provide a better understanding of the risk factors that may help to predict which patients are at increased risk for cardiotoxicity as a result of TKI therapy. In addition, there are several drugs that are in early-phase trials for the treatment of GISTs and other malignancies that would be predicted to be potentially cardiotoxic. For example, perifosine, a potent inhibitor of the protein kinase Akt, is currently in phase II trials for the treatment of imatinib-resistant GISTs.[45] A wealth of recent evidence suggests that Akt activity is indispensable for normal cardiac growth and the cardiac response to stress.[46] Thus, on mechanistic grounds, one would predict that perifosine is a potentially cardiotoxic agent.

How oncologists and cardiologists can use such information is still unclear. One must use caution in extrapolating findings from murine cardiac physiology, a system operating under lower pressures than humans and in which the resting heart rate is typically in the range of 500 beats per minute, when trying to predict the effects of pharmacologic agents on human cardiac function.[47] Similarly, preclinical toxicology studies on sedentary mice may be insufficient to exclude evidence of cardiac toxicity, especially when such agents would be mechanistically predicted to be cardiotoxic. More detailed ultrastructural analysis or addition of physiologic or pathologic stressors to preclinical drug studies may have greater yield in identifying possible cardiac toxicities preclinically. Adding to the complexity of a target-based strategy to predict cardiotoxicity is the fact that because many small-molecule TKIs exert their effects through interaction with the highly conserved ATP binding site of receptor TKs,[48] many so-called "targeted" TKIs, in fact, have inhibitory effects on a broad spectrum of TKs, introducing the possibility that an observed cardiotoxicity is attributable to off-target effects.[49] Such is the case for sunitinib, which, in addition to inhibitory effects on receptor TKs, as described in this review, seems to have broad inhibitory activity against several receptor and nonreceptor TKs (**Fig. 1**).[50] Further complicating attempts to predict which TKIs may be potentially cardiotoxic is the fact that the relevant "tyrosine kinome" that regulates normal human cardiac function is poorly understood. The human genome contains approximately 90 TKs and 43 TK-like genes.[50] Despite an understanding of some of the function of subsets of these in the cardiovascular system, including targets of GIST therapy (**Table 2**), the role of most TKs in cardiovascular function is still not known. Because some of this work proceeds through the work of molecular cardiologists studying cardiac function in

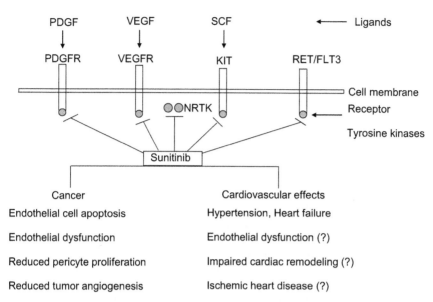

Fig.1. Sunitinib therapy–associated possible cardiotoxic effects. Flt-3, fms-like tyrosine kinase receptor-3; KIT, stem cell factor receptor; NRTK, nonreceptor tyrosine kinase; PDGFR, platelet-derived growth factor receptor; RET, RET proto-oncogene; SCF, stem cell factor; VEGFR, vascular endothelial growth factor receptor.

reductionist murine systems, the unfortunate fact remains that further understanding of the relevant tyrosine kinome of the heart may emerge, in part, through cardiotoxicities that develop as a result of novel targeted anticancer therapies.

A PRACTICAL APPROACH TO PREVENTION OF CARDIAC TOXICITY IN PATIENTS WHO HAVE GASTROINTESTINAL STROMAL TUMORS

While we await prospective studies to define the incidence of cardiotoxicity attributable to TKIs, such as imatinib and sunitinib, further and the risk factor profile

Table 2
Role of platelet-derived growth factor receptor, vascular endothelial growth factor receptor, and stem cell factor receptor in the cardiovascular system

Agent Defect	Cardiac Phenotype	Animal Model	References
KIT	Impaired cardiac remodeling and angiogenesis	MI	53–55
PDGFRα	Defects in cardiac remodeling cell proliferation and adverse cardiac remodeling	MI	56,57
PDGFRβ	Impaired muscle cell proliferation, cardiac neovessel maturity, and angiogenesis	MI	57
VEGF/VEGFR1-3	Impaired angiogenesis, increased ischemia, and impaired remodeling	MI, TAC, ischemia	58–61

Abbreviations: KIT, stem cell factor receptor; MI, myocardial infarction; TAC, transverse aortic constriction.

of patients who are at greatest risk, a practical approach to preventing cardiac complications attributable to these drugs is needed. One such approach that seems to be applicable to patients treated with sunitinib and, to a lesser extent, imatinib, is based on the recently published guidelines from the American Heart Association (AHA) for the management of congestive heart failure.[51] In this classification scheme, a new area of focus is the so-called "stage A" patient, a patient without evidence of cardiac function but at risk for heart failure. Management of such patients involves modification of risk factors that may predispose the patient to heart failure, including aggressive treatment of blood pressure, encouragement of smoking cessation, diagnosis and treatment of diabetes and hyperlipidemia, and adoption of a regular exercise program in accordance with accepted guidelines. Based on the clinical and preclinical cardiotoxicities described herein, we believe that patients treated with imatinib or sunitinib can be thought of as stage A patients, at risk for heart failure, and that application of the AHA guidelines for the stage A patient is a reasonable approach to prevent cardiac complications attributable to these remarkable new drugs.

Equally important is the development of close collaborative relations from bench to bedside between experts in oncology and experts in cardiovascular medicine.[52] Such a team approach is most likely to yield new strategies to optimize the outcomes and minimize the cardiovascular morbidity of patients who have GISTs treated with TKIs.

SUMMARY

Preclinical studies indicate that imatinib and sunitinib are potentially cardiotoxic agents. Cardiotoxicity attributable to imatinib seems to be uncommon and not associated with significant morbidity, whereas cardiotoxicity attributable to sunitinib seems to be more frequent and more severe. Further prospective clinical trials are needed to define the incidence and clinical course of TKIs used in the treatment of GISTs more accurately. In addition, the differential cardiotoxicity of sunitinib, imatinib, and other TKIs may relate to their differential target profiles. This is clearly an interdisciplinary issue; therefore, close interaction between oncologists, cardiologists, and basic research scientists is important in the understanding of TKI-mediated cardiotoxicity and the development of cardiovascular disease management strategies.

REFERENCES

1. Benjamin RS, Wiernik PH, Bachur NR. Adriamycin: a new effective agent in the therapy of disseminated sarcomas. Med Pediatr Oncol 1975;1(1):63–76.
2. Lefrak EA, Pitha J, Rosenheim S, et al. A clinicopathologic analysis of Adriamycin cardiotoxicity. Cancer 1973;32(2):302–14.
3. Schwartz RG, McKenzie WB, Alexander J, et al. Congestive heart failure and left ventricular dysfunction complicating doxorubicin therapy. Seven-year experience using serial radionuclide angiocardiography. Am J Med 1987;82(6):1109–18.
4. O'Brien ME, Wigler N, Inbar M, et al. Reduced cardiotoxicity and comparable efficacy in a phase III trial of pegylated liposomal doxorubicin HCl (CAELYX/Doxil) versus conventional doxorubicin for first-line treatment of metastatic breast cancer. Ann Oncol 2004;15(3):440–9.
5. Felker GM, Thompson RE, Hare JM, et al. Underlying causes and long-term survival in patients with initially unexplained cardiomyopathy. N Engl J Med 2000;342(15):1077–84.
6. Oeffinger KC, Mertens AC, Sklar CA, et al. Chronic health conditions in adult survivors of childhood cancer. N Engl J Med 2006;355(15):1572–82.

7. Schultz-Hector S, Trott KR. Radiation-induced cardiovascular diseases: is the epidemiologic evidence compatible with the radiobiologic data? Int J Radiat Oncol Biol Phys 2007;67(1):10–8.

8. Demetri GD, van Oosterom AT, Garrett CR, et al. Efficacy and safety of sunitinib in patients with advanced gastrointestinal stromal tumour after failure of imatinib: a randomised controlled trial. Lancet 2006;368(9544):1329–38.

9. Hurwitz H, Fehrenbacher L, Novotny W, et al. Bevacizumab plus irinotecan, fluorouracil, and leucovorin for metastatic colorectal cancer. N Engl J Med 2004;350(23):2335–42.

10. Motzer RJ, Hutson TE, Tomczak P, et al. Sunitinib versus interferon alfa in metastatic renal-cell carcinoma. N Engl J Med 2007;356(2):115–24.

11. Sherbenou DW, Druker BJ. Applying the discovery of the Philadelphia chromosome. J Clin Invest 2007;117(8):2067–74.

12. Slamon DJ, Leyland-Jones B, Shak S, et al. Use of chemotherapy plus a monoclonal antibody against HER2 for metastatic breast cancer that overexpresses HER2. N Engl J Med 2001;344(11):783–92.

13. Druker BJ, Guilhot F, O'Brien SG, et al. Five-year follow-up of patients receiving imatinib for chronic myeloid leukemia. N Engl J Med 2006;355(23):2408–17.

14. Druker BJ, Talpaz M, Resta DJ, et al. Efficacy and safety of a specific inhibitor of the BCR-ABL tyrosine kinase in chronic myeloid leukemia. N Engl J Med 2001; 344(14):1031–7.

15. Force T, Krause DS, Van Etten RA. Molecular mechanisms of cardiotoxicity of tyrosine kinase inhibition. Nat Rev Cancer 2007;7(5):332–44.

16. Saglio G, Morotti A, Mattioli G, et al. Rational approaches to the design of therapeutics targeting molecular markers: the case of chronic myelogenous leukemia. Ann N Y Acad Sci 2004;1028:423–31.

17. Hynes NE, Stern DF. The biology of erbB-2/neu/HER-2 and its role in cancer. Biochim Biophys Acta 1994;1198(2–3):165–84.

18. Sparano JA. Cardiac toxicity of trastuzumab (Herceptin): implications for the design of adjuvant trials. Semin Oncol 2001;28(1 Suppl 3):20–7.

19. Crone SA, Zhao YY, Fan L, et al. ErbB2 is essential in the prevention of dilated cardiomyopathy. Nat Med 2002;8(5):459–65.

20. Ozcelik C, Erdmann B, Pilz B, et al. Conditional mutation of the ErbB2 (HER2) receptor in cardiomyocytes leads to dilated cardiomyopathy. Proc Natl Acad Sci USA 2002;99(13):8880–5.

21. Chu TF, Rupnick MA, Kerkela R, et al. Cardiotoxicity associated with tyrosine kinase inhibitor sunitinib. Lancet 2007;370(9604):2011–9.

22. Kerkela R, Grazette L, Yacobi R, et al. Cardiotoxicity of the cancer therapeutic agent imatinib mesylate. Nat Med 2006;12(8):908–16.

23. Khakoo AY, Kassiotis CM, Tannir N, et al. Heart failure associated with sunitinib malate: a multitargeted receptor tyrosine kinase inhibitor. Cancer 2008;112(11): 2500–8.

24. Park YH, Park HJ, Kim BS, et al. BNP as a marker of the heart failure in the treatment of imatinib mesylate. Cancer Lett 2006;243(1):16–22.

25. Krause DS, Van Etten RA. Tyrosine kinases as targets for cancer therapy. N Engl J Med 2005;353(2):172–87.

26. Thomas DA, Faderl S, Cortes J, et al. Treatment of Philadelphia chromosome-positive acute lymphocytic leukemia with hyper-CVAD and imatinib mesylate. Blood 2004;103(12):4396–407.

27. Yanada M, Takeuchi J, Sugiura I, et al. High complete remission rate and promising outcome by combination of imatinib and chemotherapy for newly

diagnosed BCR-ABL-positive acute lymphoblastic leukemia: a phase II study by the Japan Adult Leukemia Study Group. J Clin Oncol 2006;24(3):460–6.

28. Schermuly RT, Dony E, Ghofrani HA, et al. Reversal of experimental pulmonary hypertension by PDGF inhibition. J Clin Invest 2005;115(10):2811–21.

29. Gottardi M, Manzato E, Gherlinzoni F. Imatinib and hyperlipidemia. N Engl J Med 2005;353(25):2722–3.

30. Su EJ, Fredriksson L, Geyer M, et al. Activation of PDGF-CC by tissue plasminogen activator impairs blood-brain barrier integrity during ischemic stroke. Nat Med 2008;14(7):731–7.

31. Deininger MW, O'Brien SG, Ford JM, et al. Practical management of patients with chronic myeloid leukemia receiving imatinib. J Clin Oncol 2003;21(8):1637–47.

32. Fernandez A, Sanguino A, Peng Z, et al. An anticancer C-Kit kinase inhibitor is reengineered to make it more active and less cardiotoxic. J Clin Invest 2007; 117(12):4044–54.

33. Waning is issued on drug for leukemia. NY Times 2006. Available at: http://www. nytimes.com/2006/07/24/business/24drug.html?_r=1&scp=1&sq=imatinib%20 warning&st=cse. Accessed December 31, 2008.

34. Atallah E, Kantarjian H, Cortes J. In reply to 'Cardiotoxicity of the cancer therapeutic agent imatinib mesylate.' Nat Med 2007;13(1):14; author reply 5–6.

35. Gambacorti-Passerini C, Tornaghi L, Franceschino A, et al. In reply to 'Cardiotoxicity of the cancer therapeutic agent imatinib mesylate'. Nat Med 2007;13(1): 13–4; author reply 5–6.

36. Hatfield A, Owen S, Pilot PR. In reply to 'Cardiotoxicity of the cancer therapeutic agent imatinib mesylate'. Nat Med 2007;13(1):13; author reply 5–6.

37. Mann DL. Targeted cancer therapeutics: the heartbreak of success. Nat Med 2006;12(8):881–2.

38. Verweij J, Casali PG, Kotasek D, et al. Imatinib does not induce cardiac left ventricular failure in gastrointestinal stromal tumour patients: analysis of EORTC-ISG-AGITG study 62005. Eur J Cancer 2007;43(6):974–8.

39. Atallah E, Durand JB, Kantarjian H, et al. Congestive heart failure is a rare event in patients receiving imatinib therapy. Blood 2007;110(4):1233–7.

40. Perik PJ, Rikhof B, de Jong FA, et al. Results of plasma N-terminal pro B-type natriuretic peptide and cardiac troponin monitoring in GIST patients do not support the existence of imatinib-induced cardiotoxicity. Ann Oncol 2008;19(2): 359–61.

41. Maitland ML, Ratain MJ. Terminal ballistics of kinase inhibitors: there are no magic bullets. Ann Intern Med 2006;145(9):702–3.

42. Rock EP, Goodman V, Jiang JX, et al. Food and drug administration drug approval summary: sunitinib malate for the treatment of gastrointestinal stromal tumor and advanced renal cell carcinoma. Oncologist 2007;12(1):107–13.

43. Abrams TJ, Murray LJ, Pesenti E, et al. Preclinical evaluation of the tyrosine kinase inhibitor SU11248 as a single agent and in combination with "standard of care" therapeutic agents for the treatment of breast cancer. Mol Cancer Ther 2003;2(10):1011–21.

44. Motzer RJ, Rini BI, Bukowski RM, et al. Sunitinib in patients with metastatic renal cell carcinoma. JAMA 2006;295(21):2516–24.

45. Crul M, Rosing H, de Klerk GJ, et al. Phase I and pharmacological study of daily oral administration of perifosine (D-21266) in patients with advanced solid tumours. Eur J Cancer 2002;38(12):1615–21.

46. Dorn GW 2nd, Force T. Protein kinase cascades in the regulation of cardiac hypertrophy. J Clin Invest 2005;115(3):527–37.

47. Benjamin IJ, Schneider MD. Learning from failure: congestive heart failure in the postgenomic age. J Clin Invest 2005;115(3):495–9.
48. Peters EC, Gray NS. Chemical proteomics identifies unanticipated targets of clinical kinase inhibitors. ACS Chem Biol 2007;2(10):661–4.
49. Chen MH, Kerkela R, Force T. Mechanisms of cardiac dysfunction associated with tyrosine kinase inhibitor cancer therapeutics. Circulation 2008;118(1):84–95.
50. Fabian MA, Biggs WH 3rd, Treiber DK, et al. A small molecule-kinase interaction map for clinical kinase inhibitors. Nat Biotechnol 2005;23(3):329–36.
51. Hunt SA, Abraham WT, Chin MH, et al. ACC/AHA 2005 guideline update for the diagnosis and management of chronic heart failure in the adult: a report of the American College of Cardiology/American Heart Association Task Force on Practice Guidelines (writing committee to update the 2001 guidelines for the evaluation and management of heart failure): developed in collaboration with the American College of Chest Physicians and the International Society for Heart and Lung Transplantation: endorsed by the Heart Rhythm Society. Circulation 2005;112(12):e154–235.
52. Ewer MS, Lenihan DJ, Khakoo AY. Sunitinib-related cardiotoxicity: an interdisciplinary issue. Nat Clin Pract Cardiovasc Med 2008;5(7):364–5.
53. Cimini M, Fazel S, Zhuo S, et al. c-kit dysfunction impairs myocardial healing after infarction. Circulation 2007;116(11 Suppl):I77–82.
54. Fazel S, Cimini M, Chen L, et al. Cardioprotective c-kit+ cells are from the bone marrow and regulate the myocardial balance of angiogenic cytokines. J Clin Invest 2006;116(7):1865–77.
55. Fazel SS, Chen L, Angoulvant D, et al. Activation of c-kit is necessary for mobilization of reparative bone marrow progenitor cells in response to cardiac injury. FASEB 2008;22(3):930–40.
56. Zymek P, Bujak M, Chatila K, et al. The role of platelet-derived growth factor signaling in healing myocardial infarcts. J Am Coll Cardiol 2006;48(11):2315–23.
57. Andrae J, Gallini R, Betsholtz C. Role of platelet-derived growth factors in physiology and medicine. Genes Dev 2008;22(10):1276–312, Review.
58. Carmeliet P, Ng YS, Nuyens D, et al. Impaired myocardial angiogenesis and ischemic cardiomyopathy in mice lacking the vascular endothelial growth factor isoforms VEGF164 and VEGF188. Nat Med 1999;5:495–502.
59. Tammela T, Enholm B, Alitalo K, et al. The biology of vascular endothelial growth factors. Cardiovasc Res 2005;65(3):550–63, Review.
60. Izumiya Y, Shiojima I, Sato K, et al. Vascular endothelial growth factor blockade promotes the transition from compensatory cardiac hypertrophy to failure in response to pressure overload. Hypertension 2006;47(5):887–93.
61. Shiojima I, Sato K, Izumiya Y, et al. Disruption of coordinated cardiac hypertrophy and angiogenesis contributes to the transition to heart failure. J Clin Invest 2005;115(8):2108–18.

Ocular Side Effects Associated with Imatinib Mesylate and Perifosine for Gastrointestinal Stromal Tumor

S. Serdar Dogan, MD, Bita Esmaeli, MD*

KEYWORDS

- Gastrointestinal stromal tumor • Perifosine • Imatinib mesylate
- Ulcerative keratitis • Periorbital edema

Gastrointestinal stromal tumor (GIST) is a mesenchymal malignancy of the gastrointestinal tract. A defining characteristic of GISTs is that they have activating KIT or platelet-derived growth factor receptor (PDGFRα) mutations and, thus, overexpress KIT or PDGFRα protein.[1,2]

Although surgical resection is the preferred treatment for GIST, at the time of presentation 47% of patients have distant metastases.[3] Targeted therapy with imatinib mesylate (imatinib; ST1571; Gleevec; Novartis Pharmaceuticals, Basel, Switzerland), a selective inhibitor of the bcr-abl, c-kit, and PDGFRα tyrosine kinases, has proven to be an effective therapeutic option for patients with GIST who are not candidates for surgery. In imatinib-resistant cases, sunitinib and perifosine combined with imatinib are the treatment choices. In this article, we will review the recently described ocular side effects of GIST therapy with imatinib, perifosine, and combinations of these two drugs.

OCULAR SIDE EFFECTS OF IMATINIB MESYLATE

Imatinib has been used effectively to treat chronic myelogenous leukemia and GISTs.[4–7] It is generally well tolerated, with mild side effects. The most common

Section of Ophthalmology, Department of Head and Neck Surgery, The University of Texas M.D. Anderson Cancer Center, Unit 441, 1515 Holcombe Boulevard, Houston, TX, 77030, USA
* Corresponding author. Section of Ophthalmology, Department of Head and Neck Surgery, The University of Texas M.D. Anderson Cancer Center, Unit 1445, 1515 Holcombe Boulevard, Houston, TX, 77030.
E-mail address: besmaeli@mdanderson.org (B. Esmaeli).

Hematol Oncol Clin N Am 23 (2009) 109–114
doi:10.1016/j.hoc.2008.11.003
0889-8588/08/$ – see front matter © 2009 Elsevier Inc. All rights reserved.

reported side effects are mild to moderate nausea, myalgias, edema, fatigue, dyspepsia, diarrhea, liver function abnormalities, erythematous and pruritic skin rash, periorbital edema, and epiphora.[8,9]

According to the World Health Organization classification, the existence of a causal relationship between imatinib and the ocular side effects reported to date is considered certain in the case of periorbital edema; probable for epiphora; possible for extraocular muscle palsy, ptosis, and blepharoconjunctivitis; and unlikely for glaucoma, papilledema, retinal hemorrhage, photosensitivity, abnormal vision, and increased intraocular pressure.[9–11]

Periorbital edema is the most common ocular side effect associated with imatinib. In a multicenter randomized trial designed to evaluate imatinib in patients with GIST, periorbital edema occurred in 74.1% of the patients.[7] A retrospective study of a case series of 104 patients treated with imatinib at the Oregon Health Science Center found that 73 patients (70%) experienced periorbital edema and 19 patients (18%) experienced epiphora. The imatinib dose had a mean value of 407.5 mg [60], and periorbital edema occurred with a mean value of 68 days [48] after the start of therapy. The patients who received more than 400 mg/day of imatinib had a higher rate of periorbital edema, suggesting that periorbital edema, due to imatinib, is dose dependent. The time of periorbital edema onset was not significantly different between patients who received more than 400 mg/day and patients who received lower doses. Twenty-nine percent of the patients with periorbital edema had concomitant peripheral edema.[9]

Histopathologic findings from the surgical debulking of periorbital tissues in a patient who developed severe periorbital edema while receiving imatinib revealed that the dermal dendrocytes, which are abundant in periocular skin, expressed c-kit and PDGFR tyrosine kinases, which are molecular targets for imatinib.[10] Dermal dendrocytes are bone marrow-derived cells that are found in normal human skin. They are distributed within the papillary dermis and underneath the dermal-epidermal junction; around superficial blood vessels, where they are associated with mast cells; and within the reticular dermis. Dermal dendrocytes may have a function in tissue repair and hemostasis, antigen presentation, and initiation of primary T–cell-mediated immune responses. They may also interact with mast cells and promote mast cell degranulation.[12,13] The expression in this patient of PDGFR tyrosine kinase in dermal dendrocytes, which are the predominant cell population in the periorbital soft tissues, suggests a possible role for dermal dendrocytes in the development of periorbital edema in patients receiving imatinib. Signaling through PDGF-β receptors increased interstitial fluid pressure in the dermis of rodents, and treatment with imatinib has been shown to decrease interstitial hypertension and increase the transport of certain molecules from capillaries to the interstitium.[14,15] Inhibition of the PDGFR on dermal dendrocytes in the periorbital skin may be the mechanism responsible for the localized edema that occurs in the periorbital soft tissues in response to imatinib. Compared with other sites in the body, the orbit may have anatomic features that make it more susceptible to collection of fluid. Collagenous septal attachments lie between the lower eyelid skin and the inferior orbital wall, forming a closed space where fluid can be trapped. Lymphatic drainage from the orbit is not as well developed as drainage from other sites. The bony orbit and its contents lack lymphatic channels, and lymphatic drainage from the periorbital region is limited to the superficial channels on the eyelid skin and conjunctiva.[16,17]

Ocular side effects in patients treated with imatinib are more severe in patients with predisposing factors (hypertension and myopia) and patients who receive high doses (600–800 mg/day). The majority of patients who develop periorbital edema have mild edema and do not require treatment. Diuretic therapy may be administered in patients with moderate to severe periorbital edema. Hydrochlorothiazide can act by reducing the blood pressure and sodium retention, which reduces the volume of extracellular fluid.[18] Although several hundred patients with GIST have been treated with imatinib at the authors' institution, to date they have not encountered any patient with GIST treated with imatinib whose periorbital edema was severe enough to require surgical debulking. The authors have encountered only one patient with such severe periorbital edema secondary to imatinib—a patient with chronic myelogenous leukemia (**Fig. 1**). In this patient, severe lower eyelid edema and festoons were causing visual obstruction. This patient was previously reported by the authors' group.[10]

Epiphora is the second most common ocular side effect associated with imatinib. The mechanism underlying epiphora as a result of imatinib is probably multifactorial. Conjunctival chemosis due to fluid retention can lead to ocular-surface irritation and overproduction of tears. Lacrimal pump dysfunction due to periorbital edema and blockage of the puncta by conjunctivochalasis can lead to epiphora. Epiphora associated with imatinib is usually improved with the use of diuretics and a short pulse of topical steroids.[9] Secretion of medication in the tear film might lead to canalicular stenosis and epiphora;[19] however, to the authors' knowledge, no study has demonstrated secretion of imatinib in the tear film.

Other reported ocular side effects associated with imatinib include increased intraocular pressure, glaucoma, recurrent retinal and conjunctival hemorrhage, optic neuritis, and cystoid macular edema following phacoemulsification surgery.[9,19–22] Conjunctival hemorrhage may be related to increased retention of fluid in the subconjunctival space. The conjunctiva is rich in c-kit-positive mast cells, inhibition of which by imatinib may be responsible for increased exposure of conjunctival mucosa to injuries.[23] In all reported cases, conjunctival hemorrhage resolved spontaneously without any systemic or local therapy. A single case of optic neuritis causing rapid loss of vision associated with imatinib has been reported in a patient with chronic myelogenous leukemia. The vision loss in this patient was reversed with the use of systemic steroids and discontinuation of imatinib.[21]

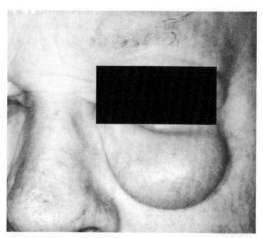

Fig. 1. Severe periorbital edema in a patient with chronic myelogenous leukemia treated with imatinib mesylate. He required surgical debulking of his lower eyelid edema to improve his visual function. (*From* Esmaeli B, Diba R, Ahmadi MA, et al. Periorbital oedema and epiphora as ocular side effects of imatinib mesylate (Gleevac). Eye 2004;18:760-2; with permission.)

OCULAR SIDE EFFECTS ASSOCIATED WITH PERIFOSINE

Most cases of GIST eventually develop resistance to imatinib.[24] Protein kinase B, a protein associated with tumor survival and growth, is activated in 10% to 50% of GISTs by phosphorylation. Protein kinase B activation is thought to promote development of resistance to imatinib by inhibiting apoptosis. Perifosine (octadecyl-[1, 1dimethyl-4-piperidylio]phosphate), a synthetic alkylphospholipid that inhibits protein kinase B activation,[25] can decrease resistance to imatinib. Perifosine, in combination with imatinib, is currently being studied in phase II clinical trials for treatment of GIST that is resistant or refractory to imatinib monotherapy. Adverse effects associated with perifosine include nausea, vomiting, diarrhea, fatigue, renal insufficiency manifesting as increased creatinine levels, and hypercalcemia.[25]

The authors have reported five patients in whom paralimbal corneal infiltration and peripheral corneal thinning developed after combination therapy with perifosine and imatinib.[26] The interval from the start of combination therapy to diagnosis of ulcerative keratitis ranged from 1 to 3 months. Two of the five patients were receiving perifosine 100 mg daily in two doses of 50 mg each. The other three patients were receiving perifosine 900 mg per week. Each patient received perifosine orally. Topical and systemic steroids, along with topical antibiotic coverage and lubrication, were the effective treatment for ulcerative keratitis in these patients.[26] Withdrawal of perifosine also helped with the ocular symptoms.

The corneal findings in these patients were most consistent with a form of peripheral ulcerative keratitis, resembling a Mooren's ulcer or other type of autoimmune keratitis (**Fig. 2**). In three of the five patients, ulcerative keratitis abated on withdrawal of perifosine and did not recur when patients were restarted on imatinib-based alternative chemotherapy without perifosine, suggesting that perifosine by itself, or in combination with imatinib, may be the cause of this ocular side effect. The mechanism underlying development of ulcerative keratitis associated with perifosine is unclear. Given that the appearance of the cornea in patients with this condition is similar to the appearance of the cornea in other forms of autoimmune keratopathy and given that the cases of ulcerative keratitis in the authors' series responded to topical steroid therapy, the authors hypothesize that either perifosine, or the combination of perifosine with imatinib, induces an autoimmune reaction in the cornea. The ulcerative keratitis associated with perifosine is reversible if detected and treated early.

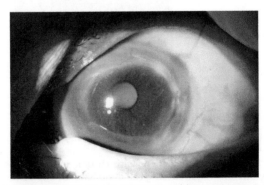

Fig. 2. Peripheral ring-shaped ulcerative keratitis, resembling a Mooren's ulcer, or other type of autoimmune keratitis, in a patient who was treated with perifosine in combination with imatinib.

SUMMARY

Two important new drugs used in treatment of GIST in recent years, imatinib mesylate and perifosine, are associated with treatable and reversible ocular side effects. Early recognition and appropriate treatment of ulcerative keratitis associated with perifosine is important to prevent sight-threatening complications.

REFERENCES

1. Fletcher CD, Berman JJ, Corless C, et al. Diagnosis of gastrointestinal stromal tumors: a consensus approach. Hum Pathol 2002;33(5):459–65.
2. Qiu FH, Ray P, Brown K, et al. Primary structure of c-kit: relationship with the CSF-1/PDGF receptor kinase family–oncogenic activation of c-kit involves deletion of extracellular domain and C terminus. EMBO J. 1988;7(4):1003–11.
3. DeMatteo RP, Lewis JJ, Leung D, et al. Two hundred gastrointestinal stromal tumors: recurrence patterns and prognostic factors for survival. Ann Surg 2000; 231(1):51–8.
4. Druker BJ, Talpaz M, Resta DJ, et al. Efficacy and safety of a specific inhibitor of the BCR-ABL tyrosine kinase in chronic myeloid leukemia. N Engl J Med 2001; 344(14):1031–7.
5. Heinrich MC, Griffith DJ, Druker BJ, et al. Inhibition of c-kit receptor tyrosine kinase activity by STI 571, a selective tyrosine kinase inhibitor. Blood 2000; 96(3):925–32.
6. van Oosterom AT, Judson I, Verweij J, et al. Safety and efficacy of imatinib (STI571) in metastatic gastrointestinal stromal tumours: a phase I study. Lancet 2001;358(9291):1421–3.
7. Demetri GD, von Mehren M, Blanke CD, et al. Efficacy and safety of imatinib mesylate in advanced gastrointestinal stromal tumors. N Engl J Med 2002;347(7): 472–80.
8. Druker BJ, Sawyers CL, Kantarjian H, et al. Activity of a specific inhibitor of the BCR-ABL tyrosine kinase in the blast crisis of chronic myeloid leukemia and acute lymphoblastic leukemia with the Philadelphia chromosome. N Engl J Med 2001; 344(14):1038–42 [Erratum in: N Engl J Med 2001 Jul 19;345(3):232].
9. Fraunfelder FW, Solomon J, Druker BJ, et al. Ocular side-effects associated with imatinib mesylate (Gleevec). J Ocul Pharmacol Ther. 2003;19(4):371–5.
10. Esmaeli B, Prieto VG, Butler CE, et al. Severe periorbital edema secondary to STI571 (Gleevec). Cancer 2002;95(4):881–7.
11. Esmaeli B, Diba R, Ahmadi MA, et al. Periorbital edema and epiphora as ocular side effects of imatinib mesylate (Gleevec). Eye 2004;18:760–2.
12. Banchereau J, Steinman RM. Dendritic cells and the control of immunity. Nature 1998;392(6673):245–52.
13. Sueki H, Whitaker D, Buchsbaum M, et al. Novel interactions between dermal dendrocytes and mast cells in human skin. Implications for hemostasis and matrix repair. Lab Invest 1993;69(2):160–72.
14. Heuchel R, Berg A, Tallquist M, et al. Platelet-derived growth factor beta receptor regulates interstitial fluid homeostasis through phosphatidylinositol-3' kinase signaling. Proc Natl Acad Sci U S A 1999;96(20):11410–5.
15. Pietras K, Ostman A, Sjöquist M, et al. Inhibition of platelet-derived growth factor receptors reduces interstitial hypertension and increases transcapillary transport in tumors. Cancer Res 2001;61(7):2929–34.
16. Koornneef L. Orbital septa: anatomy and function. Ophthalmology 1979;86(5): 876–80.

17. Kikkawa DO, Lemke BN. Applied anatomy of the eyelids, lacrimal system, and orbit. Curr Opin Ophthalmol 1991;2:568–72.

18. Breccia M, Gentilini F, Cannella L, et al. Ocular side effects in chronic myeloid leukemia patients treated with imatinib. Leuk Res 2008;32(7):1022–5.

19. Esmaeli B, Ahmadi MA, Rivera E, et al. Docetaxel secretion in tears: association with lacrimal drainage obstruction. Arch Ophthalmol 2002;120:1180–2.

20. Radaelli F, Vener C, Ripamonti F, et al. Conjunctival hemorrhagic events associated with imatinib mesylate. Int J Hematol 2007;86(5):390–3.

21. Govind Babu K, Attili VS, Bapsy PP, et al. Imatinib-induced optic neuritis in a patient of chronic myeloid leukemia. Int Ophthalmol 2007;27(1):43–4.

22. Masood I, Negi A, Dua HS. Imatinib as a cause of cystoid macular edema following uneventful phacoemulsification surgery. J Cataract Refract Surg 2005; 31(12):2427–8.

23. Stahl JL, Cook EB, Graziano FM, et al. Human conjunctival mast cells: expression of Fc epsilonRI, c-kit, ICAM-1, and IgE. Arch Ophthalmol 1999;117(4):493–7.

24. Joensuu H. Second line therapies for the treatment of gastrointestinal stromal tumor. Curr Opin Oncol 2007;19(4):353–8.

25. Kondapaka SB, Singh SS, Dasmahapatra GP, et al. Perifosine, a novel alkylphospholipid, inhibits protein kinase B activation. Mol Cancer Ther 2003;2(11): 1093–103.

26. Shome D, Trent J, Espandar L, et al. Ulcerative keratitis in gastrointestinal stromal tumor patients treated with perifosine. Ophthalmology 2008;115(3):483–7.

Hepatic Resection for Gastrointestinal Stromal Tumor Liver Metastases

Stephane Zalinski, MD, Martin Palavecino, MD, Eddie K. Abdalla, MD*

KEYWORDS

- Gastrointestinal stromal tumor • Liver metastasis
- Liver resection • Tyrosine kinase inhibitor • Imatinib
- Extended hepatectomy • Liver volumetry
- Portal vein embolization

Gastrointestinal stromal tumors (GISTs) are the most common mesenchymal tumors of the gastrointestinal tract. Immunohistochemical reactivity for KIT (CD117) is found in more than 90% of GIST cases, most often as a result of mutations in KIT, or less commonly, platelet-derived growth factor receptor-α (PDGFRα) genes.[1] These mutations lead to constitutive activation of tyrosine kinase receptors, a key element of oncogenesis in this disease. Discovery of imatinib mesylate (Gleevec; Novartis Pharmaceuticals, Basel, Switzerland), an inhibitor of KIT and PDGFRα tyrosine kinases, led to a new era in the treatment of GISTs with tyrosine kinase inhibitors (TKIs).[2,3] Response rates have been reported in up to 76% of patients who have GISTs treated with imatinib;[4] however, complete response (CR) is rare, and at least half of patients develop resistance to imatinib after approximately 2 years of treatment, likely as a result of acquisition of a secondary KIT or PDGFRα mutation.[5–7]

Up to 40% of patients who undergo complete resection of GIST primaries have recurrence[8–10] within a median time ranging from 18 to 24 months.[11] In addition, recurrence after a prolonged disease-free survival (>5 years) has been reported. Among those who have recurrence, the peritoneum and the liver are the most common metastatic sites, and patients with recurrence who are referred for evaluation have a resectable disease in 26% to 30% of cases. It is estimated from available data that the liver is a site of recurrence in most of those who are referred with recurrence after resection (67% in one series),[12] although actual rates of recurrence are difficult to define because they are based on data accrued from small and inhomogeneous

Department of Surgical Oncology, University of Texas, M.D. Anderson Cancer Center, 1515 Holcombe Boulevard, Unit 444, Houston, TX 77030, USA
* Corresponding author.
E-mail address: eabdalla@mdanderson.org (E.K. Abdalla).

Hematol Oncol Clin N Am 23 (2009) 115–127
doi:10.1016/j.hoc.2008.11.001
0889-8588/08/$ – see front matter © 2009 Elsevier Inc. All rights reserved.

series,[9,13–17] and referral patterns may have an impact on assessment of incidence and resectability of recurrent disease.

Available data that address GIST liver metastases (LMs) specifically are quite consistent and show that complete resection yields good outcomes (**Table 1**). Before the imatinib era, GISTs were treated like leiomyosarcomas metastatic to the liver; they were resistant to systemic or locoregional chemotherapy, and thus were resected when technically feasible. The 5-year overall survival rate after resection of sarcoma LMs in general was reported to be approximately 30%.[9,16,18] As a comparison, patients who had advanced disease and were not amenable to surgical resection reached a median survival time of approximately 1.5 years, and 5-year survival was rarely achieved.[19,20]

As for other solid-tumor LMs, combining systemic therapy (in this case, TKIs) with locoregional therapy (hepatic resection) is an attractive approach. Several combined approaches have been proposed. Based on the finding that most patients become resistant to imatinib, Haller and colleagues[21] recently advocated that treated patients should be considered for surgery when a "stagnation of tumor shrinkage" is observed, a "treat and wait for resistance" approach. A "neoadjuvant" approach, proposed by Gold and DeMatteo[22] and DeMatteo,[23] is to proceed to surgery within 6 months after initiation of the treatment, because the optimal imatinib response is generally observed within that time frame.[24] Finally, in patients who are not candidates for resection after adequate treatment with a TKI, the concept of "debulking"[25] has been proposed.

To frame the discussion of hepatic resection for GIST LMs, three areas are addressed. First, a general discussion of patient selection, patient preparation, and outcomes for liver resection (including major liver resection) is critical. Second, analysis of relevant data regarding oncologic outcomes for resection of sarcoma LMs and GIST LMs is revealing. Third, analysis of treatment approaches that combine surgery and systemic therapy for GISTs allow the proposal for multidisciplinary-based individualized care and the development of investigational protocols designed to answer relevant clinical questions to advance the care of patients who have this disease.

Table 1
Series reporting patients who have gastrointestinal stromal tumor liver metastases undergoing surgical treatment

Series	Surgically Treated Sarcoma LMs (n)	Surgically Treated GIST LMs (n)	Median Follow-up (Months)	1-Year Survival Rate (%)	3-Year Survival Rate (%)	5-Year Survival Rate (%)	Median Survival (Months)	Recurrence (n) [%]
DeMatteo et al[9,a]	56	34	25	88	50	30	39	47 [84]
Nunobe et al[18]	—	18	35	—	64	34	36	17 [94]
Pawlik et al[16,a]	66	36	36	91	65	27	47	44 [67]

[a] Series reporting sarcoma metastatic to liver. All variables were calculated, including all sarcoma histologic findings.

HEPATIC RESECTION FOR LIVER METASTASES
Indications and Patient Preparation for Major Resection

Indications for resection of solid-tumor LMs have dramatically changed in recent years, largely as a result of a shift from emphasis on what is removed (the tumors or tumor-bearing liver) to what remains after resection (the disease-free liver remnant). Although most study in this regard arises in the setting of colorectal LMs, safety of liver resection is clearly linked to the volume and function of the liver remnant, regardless of the reason for resection.[26–28] Although the oncologic indications for hepatic resection of liver tumors vary depending on the disease, the safety and short-term outcomes are uniformly linked to the liver remnant function. Fortunately, clear recommendations exist to guide objective volumetric measurement (by CT volumetry) of the planned future liver remnant (FLR) before major or extended hepatectomy.[29] This is critical to the discussion of GIST LMs, because patients deemed from an oncologic standpoint to be candidates for liver resection can have their risk for resection objectively estimated.

The specific limits of safe resection are gradually being defined. Up to 80% of the functional liver parenchyma can be safely resected in patients with normal underlying liver, leaving a remnant liver of 20% or greater of the standardized total liver volume.[30–32] When the underlying liver is diseased, a larger proportion of the liver must remain to ensure safety: 30% or greater FLR when moderate liver disease is present and 40% or greater FLR when compensated cirrhosis is present.[29] Fortunately, GISTs most often occur in the setting of normal underlying liver; therefore, extensive resections can often be considered and performed safely in these patients.

When disease in the liver is deemed technically resectable but the liver remnant would be inadequate based on CT volumetry, preoperative portal vein embolization (PVE) can be considered. This outpatient percutaneous procedure is performed under conscious sedation by the interventional radiologist at the request of the hepatic surgeon based on remnant volume, degree of underlying liver disease, and extent of the planned hepatic (and often extrahepatic) procedures.[33] The authors have recommended that the portal veins supplying all tumor-bearing liver be systematically occluded, leading to diversion of portal flow to the disease-free FLR. Using this approach, optimal preparation for surgery occurs (FLR hypertrophy is maximized) and tumor growth does not occur. Repeat volumetry in 3 to 4 weeks allows reassessment of liver hypertrophy; if adequate, resection of the embolized (tumor-bearing) liver is safe, with excellent results. The side effects of PVE are mild and transient, and even in large series, complications of PVE have not led to unresectability of treated patients.[34] Many studies have demonstrated the clinical value of PVE before liver resection for metastatic tumors, hepatocellular carcinoma, and biliary tract cancer.[34] The authors have performed more than 280 consecutive extended resections based on these criteria, with a 1.8% 30-day mortality rate.[32]

When multiple bilateral lesions are present (which is common with GIST LMs), a carefully planned, oncologically oriented, surgically safe approach has been devised. This approach is described as two-stage hepatectomy with or without PVE.[35] The objectives of the systematic approach are to determine which patients who have extensive hepatic disease would benefit from major resection (ie, to assess oncologic suitability based on response to chemotherapy) and to prepare the patient for and to complete resection of all the disease safely (ie, to optimize safety). The first step is to treat with chemotherapy and to proceed only in those patients who respond to therapy. Next, the "first-stage" resection is performed, which entails removal of lesions in the FLR, usually by means of minor wedge resections (the primary tumor is often resected at this stage to minimize the risk for a major hepatectomy with a major extrahepatic procedure). PVE is performed if needed based on CT volumetry, and second-stage major resection is then performed to clear remaining disease only if adequate liver hypertrophy occurs and only if the patient has recovered well from the first operation. Advantages of this approach include the common need for resection of the primary GIST in combination with treatment of GIST LMs (when major hepatic resection is not thought to be safe in combination with an extensive resection for the primary, the primary tumor resection can be performed at the time of the more minor first-stage hepatectomy, followed at an interval by major hepatectomy) and the fact that this approach maintains the objectives of therapy by enabling complete resection of disease while maximizing safety for the patient. With the advent of imatinib therapy and the common occurrence of bilateral metastases of GISTs, such a measured approach, which requires tumor response to therapy and patient response to minor surgery (and liver response to PVE if indicated), allows optimal selection of patients who have extensive disease for major hepatectomy, preserves the oncologic principles of complete resection, and allows for safe surgery.

Interpretation of Imaging and Hepatic Resection for Gastrointestinal Stromal Tumor Liver Metastases

The objectives of imaging for GIST LMs include the usual elements of disease localization and characterization but also include assessment of response; importantly, with liver surgery, definition of the anatomic associations of liver tumors with intrahepatic vascular structures; and determination of FLR volume. Imaging modalities thus must include cross-sectional imaging (CT or MRI)[36] for anatomic analysis and may also include functional imaging with[18] F-fluorodeoxyglucose (FDG) positron emission tomography (PET).

The hepatic surgeon's understanding of radiologic response to therapy is critical to accurate surgical planning. Response to tumor treatment leads, less importantly, to changes in tumor size or diameter and, more often, to changes in density, vascularity, and the cystic nature of GISTs (including GIST LMs). Thus, the commonly used World Health Organization (WHO) criteria[37] and the Response Evaluation Criteria in Solid Tumor (RECIST) criteria[38] are less useful than newer radiographic response criteria that take these morphologic changes, such as cystic transformation and tumor density, into account.[39] Functional tests, including FDG-PET, may provide additional clinically relevant information about response to therapy,[40] although tumor density may be more specific and sensitive than PET in predicting the response to targeted therapy.[39] Despite improved radiographic response criteria, however, radiographic CR does not consistently (or even frequently) predict cure of GISTs.[4] Said differently, radiologic CR does not predict pathologic CR. This finding is supported by pathologic assessment of resected specimens, which consistently contain viable tumor cells independent of radiologic CR.[4] This reality is critical to the surgeon asked to resect GIST LMs and suggests the need to resect all disease present if the objective of liver resection is complete removal of all disease. Thus, surgical planning for resection of GIST LMs is made based on anatomic imaging, with the assessment of pretreatment imaging critical to complete resection of disease.

Hepatic Resection for Sarcoma and Gastrointestinal Stromal Tumor Liver Metastases

Dematteo and colleagues[9] recently reported their retrospective experience of liver resection for sarcoma metastatic to the liver. Among 331 patients who had sarcoma metastatic to the liver, only 56 underwent grossly complete resection (R0 or R1) of hepatic disease, among whom 34 had GISTs or gastrointestinal leiomyosarcomas. Half of the patients who underwent resection required a hepatic lobectomy (hemihepatectomy) or extended lobectomy (extended hepatectomy), and there were no perioperative deaths among patients who underwent resection. Reported 1-, 3-, and 5-year actuarial survival rates were 88%, 50%, and 30%, respectively, with a median survival of 39 months, which was in contrast to a 5-year survival rate of 4% and a median survival of 12 months in patients who did not undergo resection. Factors that predicted a good outcome included the duration of the disease-free interval (DFI) from discovery of the primary sarcoma to the discovery of sarcoma LMs (5-year overall survival rate when DFI was >2 years, >50% versus 5-year survival rate <10% if DFI <2 years). These researchers not only emphasized the potential value of hepatic resection for sarcoma LMs but remarked on the value of reresection for recurrence. Of note in their study was that the outcome for the GIST LMs versus non-GIST LMs was statistically identical.[9] This work set the framework for subsequent analyses of resection for sarcoma and GIST LMs.

Pawlik and colleagues[16] reported their experience with surgical therapy for sarcoma LMs, including 66 patients who underwent hepatic resection or open radiofrequency ablation (RFA). Included were 36 GIST LMs, 18 non-GIST leiomyosarcoma LMs, and 12 unclassified sarcoma LMs. At presentation, LMs were mainly multiple (n > 3 [65%]) and bilateral (65%). Overall, 35 patients underwent resection, 18 underwent resection plus RFA, and 13 underwent RFA alone. Perioperative outcomes were good, but these researchers found that resection was significantly superior to RFA for GIST LMs because of frequent local and intrahepatic recurrence after RFA. The 1-, 3- and 5-year actuarial disease-free survival rates were 52%, 21%, and 16%, respectively. The median overall survival was 47.2 months, and the 1-, 3-, and 5-year actuarial overall survival rates were 91%, 65%, and 27%, respectively, which is similar to survival rates reported by Dematteo and colleagues.[9] In multivariate analysis, treatment with RFA (alone or in combination with resection) and surgery without adjuvant therapy were independent predictors of early relapse and death.[16] In addition, whereas most patients who had GIST LMs received imatinib therapy, the subgroup of patients who had GIST LMs treated by surgery plus imatinib seemed to have the best overall survival rate among studied groups, although this finding has yet to be assessed prospectively.

REFINING AN ONCOLOGIC APPROACH TO SURGERY

Growing understanding of clinicobiologic factors related to GIST has enhanced understanding of the prognosis for treatment. As a rational approach to resection for metastatic GISTs is devised, specifically to resection of GIST LMs, these factors come into consideration. Care must be taken not to overstate the utility of prognostic factors to determine treatment (or to exclude patients with less favorable factors from the benefits of some treatments) until further study is available, but understanding of prognostic factors is critical to development of a strategy for treatment of metastatic GISTs, specifically GIST LMs.

Gastrointestinal Stromal Tumor Biologic Features and Prognosis

First, regarding prognosis, anatomic data can be useful; primary tumor location in the stomach or omentum is associated with a better prognosis than primary tumor location in the small bowel or colorectum.[41,42] Second, morphologic data as simple as tumor size may predict overall and recurrence-free survival, and patients who have a tumor larger than 10 cm have an impaired recurrence-free survival rate[41] and a relative risk for death of 2.5.[12] Third, pathologic findings, specifically mitotic count, are used not only to predict prognosis but are included in staging for GISTs.[43] Most recently, many of these factors can now be associated with mutation analyses of KIT or PDGFRα genes; not only are specific mutations associated with anatomic tumor sites but with prognosis and response to imatinib therapy.[44]

Resistance often develops with secondary KIT or PDGFRα mutations, genomic amplification of KIT, and other incompletely defined molecular mechanisms. Among known mutations associated with GISTs, patients with exon-11 mutations have the best response to imatinib (65%);[3] those with a PDGFRα mutation seem to have a higher frequency of gastric and omental primaries and a better outcome than those with exon-11 mutations;[45] and those with an exon-9 mutation usually have a more aggressive phenotype, a small bowel or colon primary, and a lower imatinib response rate (35%–40%).[46]

Although these factors have not been assessed specifically with respect to GIST LMs but rather with respect to metastatic GISTs in general, they are likely to be important as more systematic approaches to GIST LMs are devised. It is worthwhile to reiterate that prognostic factors do not alone exclude a potential benefit to aggressive treatment, including surgery, because results from surgery, even in patients with a "poor prognosis," is potentially good, reiterating the need for case-by-case multidisciplinary evaluation of patients who have GIST LMs. Thus, mutation site and primary tumor location associated with a less favorable prognosis do not currently contraindicate resection of subsequently or synchronously discovered GIST LMs. Clinical trials may need to stratify for these factors to clarify their impact on the outcome of patients who have completely resected GIST LMs.

MULTIMODALITY THERAPY FOR GASTROINTESTINAL STROMAL TUMOR PRIMARY AND SYNCHRONOUS GASTROINTESTINAL STROMAL TUMOR LIVER METASTASES

A 50-year-old man was recently referred to the authors' center for a gastric GIST with synchronous LMs. His performance status was depressed as a result of an uncomfortable abdominal mass occupying most of the left and middle abdomen and by early satiety with weight loss of approximately 10 kg. Abdominal CT (**Fig. 1**A) revealed a large, irregular, hypervascular tumor applied to the greater curvature of the stomach, spleen, pancreas, and colon and extending under the lower pole of the left kidney. The tumor was well circumscribed and centrally necrotic. Two liver lesions compatible with metastases were seen measuring 15 × 12 cm and 2 × 3 cm in diameter. Both were anatomically confined to the right liver. Prereferral biopsy of the larger liver mass confirmed metastatic GIST, positive for CD34 and C-Kit. Upper endoscopy showed no intraluminal abnormality. Because of the patient's impaired performance status and need for multiorgan resection, imatinib therapy was initiated (400 mg/d). Restaging revealed a response, and his performance status steadily improved. Surgery was proposed after 4 months of therapy, but the patient refused. Imatinib therapy was continued, and a complete radiologic response was reported with cystic transformation of the primary and liver lesions (see **Fig. 1**B).

After almost 1 year of imatinib therapy, the patient agreed to surgery. Exploration revealed a 14-cm tumor involving only 3 cm of the greater curvature of the stomach, which could be separated from the spleen and pancreas but also involved a portion of the splenic flexure of colon. The lesion was resected with a small portion of the stomach and colon en bloc. Pathologic analysis of the primary tumor revealed a 14-cm gastric primary mass adherent to the colon, with negative margins. At the same operation, a right hepatectomy was performed. Two masses were found within

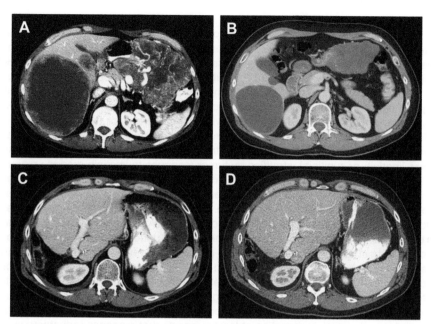

Fig. 1. A 50-year-old male patient with history of abdominal pain. (*A*) CT revealed a large heterogeneous abdominal mass contiguous with the greater curvature of the stomach and two liver tumors, with the larger measuring 15 cm. GIST LMs were proved by biopsy. Performance and nutritional status was poor at diagnosis. (*B*) After a 1-year treatment with imatinib, a substantial decrease in the size of the gastric tumor and cystic transformation of the LMs occurred, with marked improvement in the performance status. (*C*) Patient underwent an uneventful resection of the abdominal mass with a partial gastrectomy and a right hepatectomy. The pathologic analysis of the primary and liver tumors revealed a GIST primary and metastases with marked treatment effect but with viable cells in all resected tumors; molecular analysis identified a deletion in exon 11 of the KIT gene. (*D*) Two-year follow-up CT shows no evidence of recurrent disease.

the liver measuring 11 and 2.4 cm, respectively. The primary tumor and the LMs showed a marked response to treatment with imatinib but with viable cells in the primary and metastatic lesions. The hepatic parenchymal transection margin was negative for tumor. Molecular analysis of the primary and LMs revealed an exon-11 deletion in the KIT gene. The postoperative course was uncomplicated, and the patient was discharged the eighth postoperative day. Gleevec was restarted; 2 years after surgery, the patient remains free of disease (see **Fig. 1**C and D).

Surgery and Chemical (Biologic) Therapy

This case highlights several benefits to the combination of TKI therapy and surgery (see **Fig. 1**C and D). The patient's performance and nutritional status improved; the lesions downsized, facilitating surgery and organ preservation; and surgery complimented the TKI therapy by removing remaining viable tumor, ostensibly before mutation occurred. The proper duration of preoperative therapy, whether postoperative therapy should be provided, and the duration of therapy are all unanswered questions raised by such a case, however.

Historically, GISTs have been described to be resistant to any regimen of radiotherapy or chemotherapy.[12,47–49] With a reported response rate of less than 10%,[50] irrespective of the regimen used, no chemotherapy was found efficient enough to improve patients' prognosis and surgery was the only recognized treatment.[12,19,51] The combination of systemic and local regional therapy is an emergent field of clinical research,[52–55] and as with other solid-tumor LMs, there is great interest in combining chemotherapy with surgery; however, less is known about the importance of the response to imatinib with regard to the outcome from liver resection for GIST LMs. As for other solid-tumors treated with chemotherapy, the initial response to imatinib is gratifying, but most patients eventually progress to therapy, reasserting the potential advantage of the combination of surgery with chemotherapy for GISTs.

Raut and colleagues[55] assessed the role of surgery in patients who had an unresectable primary or metastatic GIST treated with targeted therapy (TKI; in this study, imatinib or sunitinib), stratified by tumor response to imatinib graded primarily by radiologic assessment. Patients were considered to have stable disease (defined as initially unresectable, converted to resectable after TKI therapy), limited disease progression (multifocal disease with some progression on TKI but fully resectable), and generalized progression (multifocal, not completely resectable). The result was as expected; that is, those responding to therapy and undergoing complete resection had the highest overall 1-year survival rate (95%) and lowest rate of progression at 1 year (20%) of the three groups. Those with disease progressing on therapy but who underwent complete resection (limited disease resection group) had an intermediate outcome, and those with unresectable progressive disease (generalized progression) who underwent incomplete resection did poorly. Comparison of the first two groups that underwent complete resection at least suggests that response to therapy, even in patients who present with initially unresectable disease, is a good "biologic" sign and that those patients derive a durable benefit from surgery. The somewhat unrelated finding that progression on therapy followed by incomplete surgery leads to a poor outcome (0% 1-year survival rate) has less significance, because the role for complete resection of progressing disease was not answered by that study.[55] These findings, well known for other disease types, do, however, suggest the value of tumor response in selection of patients who have GISTs for surgery. No such study has been done for GIST LMs; however, currently, there seems to be no role for incomplete resection of GIST LMs, particularly in the face of progressive disease.

Given high response rates (ranging from 50%–76%)[4,56] for patients who have GIST metastases treated with TKI, administration of imatinib to downsize GIST LMs in patients otherwise not deemed to be candidates for resection is an attractive approach, because a similar approach has been successful with good long-term outcomes in other diseases.[57] In addition to resectability, tumor shrinkage may enable safer surgery with a decreased risk for intraperitoneal rupture and tumor dissemination during tumor mobilization. With regard to liver resection, downsizing tumors may allow parenchymal preservation. From an oncologic standpoint, response (downsizing or cystic transformation) may suggest "favorable" biology, could be shown to enhance patient selection for hepatectomy, and may lead to improved performance status enabling major surgery. Importantly, the significance of radiologic response should not be overinterpreted, because pathologic CR is rare (5%–10%)[4,24,52,56,58] and virtually all patients treated with imatinib ultimately develop resistance.[11] Thus, although treatment with response may enhance selection for resection, there are no data yet to support replacement of resection with targeted therapy.

Secondary resistance to treatment occurs at a median of 20 to 24 months after treatment initiation,[59] but most response occurs within the first few months, which raises the question as to the optimal timing for surgery. Thus, based on clinical data for outcome based on response, the treat and wait for resistance approach[21] seems less biologically attractive than the neoadjuvant approach.[22,23]

Given the potential benefit of TKIs in most patients to downsize disease (thereby decreasing the extent of surgery), improve performance status (improve tolerance to aggressive treatment), and possibly improve selection for surgery (better results with responsive disease?), in addition to the favorable toxicity profile for TKIs, most patients who have resectable or unresectable GISTs (LMs) may be best served with TKI treatment followed by surgery. For patients who are candidates for resection, approximately 6 months of preoperative treatment seems adequate; for patients who are not candidates for resection, resection can be considered as soon as downsizing allows complete resection (not waiting for mutation and resistance). Adjuvant postoperative treatment can then be considered.

Thus, it is clear that complete removal of GIST LMs provides a significant possibility for long-term survival, but feasible clinical trials should be devised. The Z9001 phase III trial of the American College of Surgeons Oncology Group (ACOSOG), whose aim was to clarify which patients who have resected primary GISTs may benefit from adjuvant therapy with imatinib mesylate, demonstrated an improvement in recurrence-free survival among patients receiving imatinib. Based on these findings, a randomized trial comparing patients undergoing GIST LM resection with or without adjuvant imatinib could be envisioned using known prognostic molecular factors for stratification to answer the question of benefit to postoperative imatinib, with the hope of a result similar to the Z9001 trial. Another approach would be to study resectable GIST LMs, and to randomize to imatinib before surgery (eg, for 6 months) versus no preoperative therapy, to determine whether imatinib actually improves selection for surgery and surgical outcome. Other concepts may evolve as results of the ongoing M.D. Anderson Cancer Center trial of short-term preoperative therapy become available; that study is designed to determine if apoptosis induction or inhibition of angiogenesis are involved in the antitumor activity of imatinib in patients who have GISTs by examining patients who have resectable GISTs treated with imatinib 7, 5, or 3 days before surgery and continued 2 years after surgery. The concept of short-term induction therapy could be quite attractive from a biologic and patient care standpoint, particularly with regard to patients who have resectable GIST LMs.

SUMMARY

The optimal therapy for GIST LMs is complete resection. The combination of resection with TKI therapy is likely to improve outcome, although the details of TKI administration, including timing (preoperative versus postoperative versus both) and duration of therapy (before or after surgery), have yet to be defined. Based on current data, it seems that short-duration preoperative therapy (eg, 6 months) may not only reduce the extent of needed surgery but allow for "biologic selection" of the best candidates for surgery, especially when extensive procedures are planned (as with other solid-tumor LMs). Waiting for progression on treatment is a less attractive option, because the development of resistance by means of mutation may have a negative impact on long-term outcome. Use of advanced techniques for hepatic resection (eg, two-stage hepatectomy, extended hepatectomy), attention to remnant liver volume, and use of preoperative preparation (PVE) should increase the population of patients who have GIST LMs and can undergo complete resection of disease.

REFERENCES

1. Joensuu H. Gastrointestinal stromal tumor (GIST). Ann Oncol 2006;17(Suppl 10): x280–6.

2. Joensuu H, Roberts PJ, Sarlomo-Rikala M, et al. Effect of the tyrosine kinase inhibitor STI571 in a patient with a metastatic gastrointestinal stromal tumor. N Engl J Med 2001;344(14):1052–6.

3. van Oosterom AT, Judson I, Verweij J, et al. Safety and efficacy of imatinib (STI571) in metastatic gastrointestinal stromal tumours: a phase I study. Lancet 2001;358(9291):1421–3.

4. Scaife CL, Hunt KK, Patel SR, et al. Is there a role for surgery in patients with "unresectable" cKIT+ gastrointestinal stromal tumors treated with imatinib mesylate? Am J Surg 2003;186(6):665–9.

5. Antonescu CR, Besmer P, Guo T, et al. Acquired resistance to imatinib in gastrointestinal stromal tumor occurs through secondary gene mutation. Clin Cancer Res 2005;11(11):4182–90.

6. Chen LL, Trent JC, Wu EF, et al. A missense mutation in KIT kinase domain 1 correlates with imatinib resistance in gastrointestinal stromal tumors. Cancer Res 2004;64(17):5913–9.

7. Heinrich MC, Corless CL, Demetri GD, et al. Kinase mutations and imatinib response in patients with metastatic gastrointestinal stromal tumor. J Clin Oncol 2003;21(23):4342–9.

8. Crosby JA, Catton CN, Davis A, et al. Malignant gastrointestinal stromal tumors of the small intestine: a review of 50 cases from a prospective database. Ann Surg Oncol 2001;8(1):50–9.

9. DeMatteo RP, Shah A, Fong Y, et al. Results of hepatic resection for sarcoma metastatic to liver. Ann Surg 2001;234(4):540–7 [discussion 547–8].

10. Pierie JP, Choudry U, Muzikansky A, et al. The effect of surgery and grade on outcome of gastrointestinal stromal tumors. Arch Surg 2001;136(4): 383–9.

11. Katz SC, DeMatteo RP. Gastrointestinal stromal tumors and leiomyosarcomas. J Surg Oncol 2008;97(4):350–9.

12. DeMatteo RP, Lewis JJ, Leung D, et al. Two hundred gastrointestinal stromal tumors: recurrence patterns and prognostic factors for survival. Ann Surg 2000;231(1):51–8.

13. Adam R, Chiche L, Aloia T, et al. Hepatic resection for noncolorectal nonendocrine liver metastases: analysis of 1,452 patients and development of a prognostic model. Ann Surg 2006;244(4):524–35.

14. Elias D, Cavalcanti de Albuquerque A, Eggenspieler P, et al. Resection of liver metastases from a noncolorectal primary: indications and results based on 147 monocentric patients. J Am Coll Surg 1998;187(5):487–93.

15. Hemming AW, Sielaff TD, Gallinger S, et al. Hepatic resection of noncolorectal nonneuroendocrine metastases. Liver Transpl 2000;6(1):97–101.

16. Pawlik TM, Vauthey JN, Abdalla EK, et al. Results of a single-center experience with resection and ablation for sarcoma metastatic to the liver. Arch Surg 2006; 141(6):537–43 [discussion 543–4].

17. Schwartz SI. Hepatic resection for noncolorectal nonneuroendocrine metastases. World J Surg 1995;19(1):72–5.

18. Nunobe S, Sano T, Shimada K, et al. Surgery including liver resection for metastatic gastrointestinal stromal tumors or gastrointestinal leiomyosarcomas. Jpn J Clin Oncol 2005;35(6):338–41.

19. Perez EA, Gutierrez JC, Jin X, et al. Surgical outcomes of gastrointestinal sarcoma including gastrointestinal stromal tumors: a population-based examination. J Gastrointest Surg 2007;11(1):114–25.

20. Perez EA, Livingstone AS, Franceschi D, et al. Current incidence and outcomes of gastrointestinal mesenchymal tumors including gastrointestinal stromal tumors. J Am Coll Surg 2006;202(4):623–9.
21. Haller F, Detken S, Schulten HJ, et al. Surgical management after neoadjuvant imatinib therapy in gastrointestinal stromal tumours (GISTs) with respect to imatinib resistance caused by secondary KIT mutations. Ann Surg Oncol 2007;14(2): 526–32.
22. Gold JS, Dematteo RP. Neoadjuvant therapy for gastrointestinal stromal tumor (GIST): racing against resistance. Ann Surg Oncol 2007;14(4):1247–8.
23. DeMatteo RP. Treatment of advanced gastrointestinal stromal tumor: a marriage of targeted therapy and surgery? Ann Surg Oncol 2007;14(1):1–2.
24. Verweij J, Casali PG, Zalcberg J, et al. Progression-free survival in gastrointestinal stromal tumours with high-dose imatinib: randomised trial. Lancet 2004; 364(9440):1127–34.
25. Pantaleo MA, Di Battista M, Catena F, et al. Surgical debulking of gastrointestinal stromal tumors: is it a reasonable option after second-line treatment with sunitinib? J Cancer Res Clin Oncol 2008;134(5):625–30.
26. Farges O, Belghiti J, Kianmanesh R, et al. Portal vein embolization before right hepatectomy: prospective clinical trial. Ann Surg 2003;237(2):208–17.
27. Nagino M, Kamiya J, Nishio H, et al. Two hundred forty consecutive portal vein embolizations before extended hepatectomy for biliary cancer: surgical outcome and long-term follow-up. Ann Surg 2006;243(3):364–72.
28. Shoup M, Gonen M, D'Angelica M, et al. Volumetric analysis predicts hepatic dysfunction in patients undergoing major liver resection. J Gastrointest Surg 2003;7(3):325–30.
29. Abdalla EK, Adam R, Bilchik AJ, et al. Improving resectability of hepatic colorectal metastases: expert consensus statement. Ann Surg Oncol 2006; 13(10):1271–80.
30. Abdalla EK, Barnett CC, Doherty D, et al. Extended hepatectomy in patients with hepatobiliary malignancies with and without preoperative portal vein embolization. Arch Surg 2002;137(6):675–80 [discussion 680–1].
31. Vauthey JN, Pawlik TM, Abdalla EK, et al. Is extended hepatectomy for hepatobiliary malignancy justified? Ann Surg 2004;239(5):722–30 [discussion 730–2].
32. Vauthey JN, Palavecino M, Curley SA, et al. Re: right hepatic trisectionectomy for hepatobiliary disease: results and an appraisal of its current role. Ann Surg 2008; 248(1):138–9 [author reply 139–40].
33. Madoff DC, Hicks ME, Vauthey JN, et al. Transhepatic portal vein embolization: anatomy, indications, and technical considerations. Radiographics 2002;22(5): 1063–76.
34. Ribero D, Abdalla EK, Madoff DC, et al. Portal vein embolization before major hepatectomy and its effects on regeneration, resectability and outcome. Br J Surg 2007;94(11):1386–94.
35. Chun YS, Vauthey JN. Extending the frontiers of resectability in advanced colorectal cancer. Eur J Surg Oncol 2007;33(Suppl 2):S52–8.
36. Chun YS, Ribero D, Abdalla EK, et al. Comparison of two methods of future liver remnant volume measurement. J Gastrointest Surg 2008;12(1):123–8.
37. Miller AB, Hoogstraten B, Staquet M, et al. Reporting results of cancer treatment. Cancer 1981;47(1):207–14.
38. Therasse P, Arbuck SG, Eisenhauer EA, et al. New guidelines to evaluate the response to treatment in solid tumors. European Organization for Research and

Treatment of Cancer, National Cancer Institute of the United States, National Cancer Institute of Canada. J Natl Cancer Inst 2000;92(3):205–16.

39. Choi H, Charnsangavej C, Faria SC, et al. Correlation of computed tomography and positron emission tomography in patients with metastatic gastrointestinal stromal tumor treated at a single institution with imatinib mesylate: proposal of new computed tomography response criteria. J Clin Oncol 2007;25(13):1753–9.

40. Van den Abbeele AD, Badawi RD. Use of positron emission tomography in oncology and its potential role to assess response to imatinib mesylate therapy in gastrointestinal stromal tumors (GISTs). Eur J Cancer 2002;38(Suppl 5):S60–5.

41. Dematteo RP, Gold JS, Saran L, et al. Tumor mitotic rate, size, and location independently predict recurrence after resection of primary gastrointestinal stromal tumor (GIST). Cancer 2008;112(3):608–15.

42. Martin J, Poveda A, Llombart-Bosch A, et al. Deletions affecting codons 557–558 of the c-KIT gene indicate a poor prognosis in patients with completely resected gastrointestinal stromal tumors: a study by the Spanish Group for Sarcoma Research (GEIS). J Clin Oncol 2005;23(25):6190–8.

43. Hassan I, You YN, Shyyan R, et al. Surgically managed gastrointestinal stromal tumors: a comparative and prognostic analysis. Ann Surg Oncol 2008;15(1): 52–9.

44. Heinrich MC, Corless CL, Blanke CD, et al. Molecular correlates of imatinib resistance in gastrointestinal stromal tumors. J Clin Oncol 2006;24(29):4764–74.

45. Debiec-Rychter M, Dumez H, Judson I, et al. Use of c-KIT/PDGFRA mutational analysis to predict the clinical response to imatinib in patients with advanced gastrointestinal stromal tumours entered on phase I and II studies of the EORTC Soft Tissue and Bone Sarcoma Group. Eur J Cancer 2004;40(5):689–95.

46. Debiec-Rychter M, Sciot R, Le Cesne A, et al. KIT mutations and dose selection for imatinib in patients with advanced gastrointestinal stromal tumours. Eur J Cancer 2006;42(8):1093–103.

47. Bucher P, Villiger P, Egger JF, et al. Management of gastrointestinal stromal tumors: from diagnosis to treatment. Swiss Med Wkly 2004;134(11–12):145–53.

48. Dematteo RP, Heinrich MC, El-Rifai WM, et al. Clinical management of gastrointestinal stromal tumors: before and after STI-571. Hum Pathol 2002;33(5):466–77.

49. Rossi CR, Mocellin S, Mencarelli R, et al. Gastrointestinal stromal tumors: from a surgical to a molecular approach. Int J Cancer 2003;107(2):171–6.

50. Maluccio MA, Covey AM, Schubert J, et al. Treatment of metastatic sarcoma to the liver with bland embolization. Cancer 2006;107(7):1617–23.

51. Clary BM, DeMatteo RP, Lewis JJ, et al. Gastrointestinal stromal tumors and leiomyosarcoma of the abdomen and retroperitoneum: a clinical comparison. Ann Surg Oncol 2001;8(4):290–9.

52. Bonvalot S, Eldweny H, Pechoux CL, et al. Impact of surgery on advanced gastrointestinal stromal tumors (GIST) in the imatinib era. Ann Surg Oncol 2006;13(12):1596–603.

53. DeMatteo RP, Maki RG, Singer S, et al. Results of tyrosine kinase inhibitor therapy followed by surgical resection for metastatic gastrointestinal stromal tumor. Ann Surg 2007;245(3):347–52.

54. Gronchi A, Fiore M, Miselli F, et al. Surgery of residual disease following molecular-targeted therapy with imatinib mesylate in advanced/metastatic GIST. Ann Surg 2007;245(3):341–6.

55. Raut CP, Posner M, Desai J, et al. Surgical management of advanced gastrointestinal stromal tumors after treatment with targeted systemic therapy using kinase inhibitors. J Clin Oncol 2006;24(15):2325–31.

56. Demetri GD, von Mehren M, Blanke CD, et al. Efficacy and safety of imatinib mesylate in advanced gastrointestinal stromal tumors. N Engl J Med 2002; 347(7):472–80.
57. Adam R, Delvart V, Pascal G, et al. Rescue surgery for unresectable colorectal liver metastases downstaged by chemotherapy: a model to predict long-term survival. Ann Surg 2004;240(4):644–57.
58. Verweij J, van Oosterom A, Blay JY, et al. Imatinib mesylate (STI-571 Glivec, Gleevec) is an active agent for gastrointestinal stromal tumours, but does not yield responses in other soft-tissue sarcomas that are unselected for a molecular target. Results from an EORTC Soft Tissue and Bone Sarcoma Group phase II study. Eur J Cancer 2003;39(14):2006–11.
59. Gutierrez JC, De Oliveira LO, Perez EA, et al. Optimizing diagnosis, staging, and management of gastrointestinal stromal tumors. J Am Coll Surg 2007;205(3): 479–91 [quiz 524].

Gastrointestinal Stromal Tumor: Role of Interventional Radiology in Diagnosis and Treatment

Rony Avritscher, MD*, Sanjay Gupta, MD

KEYWORDS

- Gastrointestinal stromal tumor • Liver neoplasms, secondary
- Chemoembolization • Radiofrequency ablation
- Hepatic artery embolization

Gastrointestinal stromal tumors (GISTs) are the most common nonepithelial tumors of the gastrointestinal tract. GISTs are soft tissue sarcomas originating from the interstitial cells of Cajal, which are intestinal pacemaker cells. These are rare tumors whose true incidence is difficult to determine because only after the recent advent of specific immunohistochemical studies could GISTs be distinguished as a separate pathologic entity. A 2005 population-based study by Nilsson found the annual incidence of GISTs in Sweden to be 14.5 cases per million persons.[1] This translates into approximately 4000 to 5000 new cases in the United States annually.[2] Approximately 60% of GISTs occur in the stomach, 25% in the small intestine, and the rest in the large bowel, rectum, appendix, esophagus, and, rarely, in extra-intestinal sites.

GISTs exhibit a wide spectrum of clinical behavior; certain lesions remain stable over a period of years, whereas other GISTs rapidly progress to widespread metastatic disease.[3] Surgery remains the only potentially curative treatment for this disease. Unfortunately, GISTs typically have a high local recurrence rate. Moreover, at presentation, approximately half of these tumors have already metastasized, most commonly to the liver and peritoneum or both.[4–6]

The discovery of the Kit tyrosine kinase receptor and the development of imatinib mesylate (Gleevec; Novartis Pharma, Basel, Switzerland), a targeted molecular agent that blocks the activity of this receptor has drastically changed the management of patients with unresectable GISTs.[6] Imatinib is a tyrosine kinase inhibitor (TKI) that

Department of Diagnostic Radiology, The University of Texas M.D. Anderson Cancer Center, 1515 Holcombe Boulevard, Unit 325, Houston, TX 77030, USA
* Corresponding author.
E-mail address: rony.avritscher@mdanderson.org (R. Avritscher).

Hematol Oncol Clin N Am 23 (2009) 129–137
doi:10.1016/j.hoc.2008.11.002
0889-8588/08/$ – see front matter © 2009 Elsevier Inc. All rights reserved.

has been shown to produce a partial tumor response or tumor stabilization in 70% to 85% of patients with advanced disease.[6] With imatinib therapy, the median progression-free survival duration is in the range of 20 to 24 months, and the estimated median overall survival duration exceeds 36 months.[6] Unfortunately, approximately 15% of patients have tumors that show no response to this drug, and in a proportion of patients whose tumors do exhibit a response, resistance to the drug develops after an average of 2 years of treatment.[7] Another TKI, sunitinib malate (SU11248; Sutent, Pfizer Inc, New York, NY), has been shown to achieve antitumor responses in imatinib-refractory GISTs.[8]

Locoregional therapy using interventional radiology techniques, such as hepatic artery embolization (HAE) and hepatic artery chemoembolization (HACE), is a viable alternative for patients with hepatic metastatic disease who were not surgical candidates. This article will discuss the current role of interventional radiology in diagnosis and treatment of patients with GISTs.

INTERVENTIONAL RADIOLOGY IN THE DIAGNOSIS OF GISTS
Biopsy

The preoperative diagnosis of GIST requires a high level of suspicion and familiarity with its radiologic manifestations. Although preoperative biopsy is not recommended for resectable lesions in which there is a high suspicion of GIST, these infrequently occurring tumors are rarely diagnosed solely on the basis of imaging studies and, thus, percutaneous biopsies are often performed inadvertently.[9] Image-guided percutaneous biopsy carries the theoretic risk of rupture of the tumor capsule with peritoneal spread of disease. Endoscopic ultrasound-guided biopsy is being increasingly used for preoperative diagnosis of gastrointestinal submucosal lesions and has been shown to be safe and accurate. The diagnosis of GIST based on needle biopsy results requires an experienced pathologist. Frequently, the diagnosis cannot be reliably ascertained only from fine-needle aspirates. Thus, when percutaneous biopsy is performed, core samples must also be obtained. Immediate assessment of the biopsy samples by on-site pathologists is advisable to prevent sampling only necrotic or hemorrhagic areas of the tumor.

Despite these considerations, image-guided percutaneous biopsy of a lesion suspicious for GIST may be indicated in patients with clearly unresectable disease, or in cases where a lesion is marginally resectable and neoadjuvant chemotherapy is under consideration for the patient's treatment.[9] Biopsy may be appropriate in cases where it can potentially change the treatment, as would be the case when another diagnosis is entertained. Percutaneous biopsy is also useful for obtaining pathologic proof of metastases, thus, helping in tumor staging at initial presentation or to document spread of tumor at a later stage. Biopsy is useful for detecting residual or recurrent disease following treatment. Percutaneous biopsies are also required to obtain tissue to determine the tumor biomarkers; this is especially important as cancer therapy becomes more tailored to patients' distinct tumor biomarker profiles.

INTERVENTIONAL RADIOLOGY IN LOCOREGIONAL THERAPY FOR GISTS
Radiofrequency Ablation

The use of thermal ablation to produce necrosis in focal hepatic malignancies has been established in patients who are not otherwise candidates for surgery. However, only a few series have been published that have studied the efficacy of ablative therapies in sarcomas metastatic to the liver. In 2004, Dileo reported a series of nine patients with metastatic GIST treated with percutaneous radiofrequency ablation

(RFA) for a solitary or limited number of progressing hepatic and peritoneal lesions.[10] These patients had received imatinib for a median of 25 months before the ablation therapy. All lesions were successfully treated with no reported complications. In four patients, disease remained stable with imatinib therapy after RFA with a median follow-up of 5.8 months. In that series, one focal progressive peritoneal metastasis was also successfully treated with RFA.[10]

Pawlik and colleagues[11] reported a series with 31 patients who underwent intraoperative RFA of sarcoma metastatic to the liver. In that study, RFA alone was performed in 13 patients whose lesions were in unresectable locations. Resection of large lesions was combined with RFA of smaller lesions deemed otherwise unresectable in 18 patients. Those patients treated with RFA alone, or in combination with surgical resection, had a significantly higher rate of recurrence (90.9%) than did patients who underwent resection alone (57.1%).[11] These results indicated that patients whose disease cannot be treated with surgical resection alone have a substantially increased risk of recurrence.

In 2007, Hasegawa and colleagues[12] reported a series of three patients who had advanced GIST with focal liver progression successfully treated with RFA. Those patients remained progression-free at 8, 15, and 16 months after ablation.

RFA appears to be a viable palliative option for patients with advanced GIST who develop focal progression of liver or peritoneal disease during imatinib therapy and who are not otherwise candidates for surgical resection. Alternatively, RFA offers a potentially curative option for patients who exhibit a partial response to imatinib and have focal residual disease that is not amenable to surgical resection.

Hepatic Arterial Embolization and Chemoembolization

Liver metastases from gastrointestinal stromal tumors are generally hypervascular and derive 90% of their blood supply from the hepatic artery. This feature, combined with the facts that liver has a dual-blood supply and normal liver receives 80% of its blood supply from the portal vein, provides a good rationale for using either hepatic arterial embolization (HAE) or chemoembolization (HACE) to treat these metastases. HAE involves injection of an embolic agent into the vessel supplying the tumor and results in selective tumor ischemia by reducing the blood supply to the tumor. HACE is a combination of local intra-arterial delivery of chemotherapy and arterial embolization. In addition to inducing selective tumor ischemia, HACE provides a much higher concentration of chemotherapeutic agent in the tumor as compared with systemic administration.[13–15] Also, injection of an embolic agent markedly prolongs the dwell time of the chemotherapy in the tumor. Finally, only a small amount of the drug reaches the systemic circulation, minimizing systemic toxicity even at high doses.[13–15]

A preliminary arteriography of the celiac axis and superior mesenteric artery is performed to evaluate the arterial supply to the liver and to ensure the patency of the portal vein (**Fig. 1**). After the initial diagnostic arteriogram, the selected hepatic artery is catheterized with a 5-F catheter or a coaxially advanced microcatheter. For HAE, the embolic agent is injected under fluoroscopic control until stasis or substantial slowing of blood flow is achieved. However, there is no consensus on the best embolization protocol for HACE procedure. One of the most common techniques, routinely used for hepatocellular carcinomas, involves injection of chemotherapeutic agents emulsified with ethiodized oil followed by embolization with particulate agents.[16] Although some interventional radiologists use the same technique for metastatic liver disease also,[16,17] others prefer the nonoily chemoembolization for metastatic liver disease.[18–22] For nonoily chemoembolization, the chemotherapeutic agent can be mixed with the embolic agent and injected as a bolus in aliquots of 1- to -2 mL, or

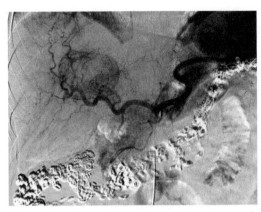

Fig. 1. Celiac angiogram in patient with metastatic GIST shows a hypervascular tumor supplied by branches of the right hepatic artery. This tumor was treated with hepatic artery chemoembolization.

the selected chemotherapeutic agent is administered first followed by the embolic material. Another technique involves initial injection of a small amount of embolic agent into the artery until slowing of flow is noted, followed by administration of the chemotherapeutic agent.[20] This is followed by more particulate embolization to achieve stasis of blood flow.

In patients with bilobar disease, embolization of the whole liver in a single treatment session is generally avoided because of the risk of prolonged postembolization syndrome or liver failure. Only one lobe of the liver is subjected to embolization during each treatment session; generally, the hepatic lobe with the greatest tumor burden is treated first. To avoid liver failure in patients with extensive (>75% liver parenchyma replaced with tumor) liver involvement, only a small portion of the liver lobe is subjected to embolization during each session. Additional HACE procedures are performed with the goal of treating the entire liver. The timing of subsequent HACE procedures is generally determined by the patient's physical condition, tumor status, response to initial embolization, and ability to tolerate the procedure.[20]

Patients with severe anaphylactoid reactions to iodinated contrast media, uncorrected coagulopathy, or severe renal insufficiency cannot be treated with HACE. Patients with portal vein occlusion and no hepatopetal flow or hepatic encephalopathy are also excluded. Extensive liver involvement and mildly abnormal liver functions (serum albumin level <3 g/dL, aspartate transaminase level >100 U/L, lactate dehydrogenase level >425 IU/mL, serum bilirubin level >2 mg/dL) indicate an increased risk of liver failure after HACE.[16,20,23] If several of these factors are combined, the risk of liver failure may be unacceptable.

HAE and HACE have been employed in the treatment of liver-dominant metastatic GIST. Maluccio and colleagues[24] reported a series of 24 patients who had metastatic sarcoma treated with bland HAE, including 16 patients with GIST. The embolization was performed with polyvinyl alcohol (PVA) microspheres (Cook Inc., Bloomington, IN) or trisacryl microspheres (Embosphere, Wayland, MA). No chemotherapy or iodized oil was used in combination with the embolic material. The overall survival rates for the 24 patients were 62% at 1 year, 41% at 2 years, and 29% at 3 years, with an overall median survival of 24 months. The seven patients who remained alive for more than 4 years after the initial embolization had metastatic GIST. Complications were observed after five (11%) embolizations. Most of the patients included in this study were enrolled before the advent of imatinib.

Four studies have investigated the use of HACE for locoregional therapy of liver-dominant metastatic GIST. In the initial report in 1991, Mavligit and colleagues[21] reported tumor regression in two patients with gastrointestinal leiomyosarcoma after HACE with cisplatin and PVA followed by hepatic arterial infusion of vinblastine. In 1995, Mavligit and his group[22] published a series of 14 patients with gastrointestinal leiomyosarcoma metastatic to the liver treated with HACE using the combination of cisplatin and PVA followed by arterial infusion of vinblastine. Those investigators reported a 70% radiologic response rate with an overall median survival duration of 12 months after an average of two procedures. In 2001, Rajan and colleagues[25] published their experience with TACE for the treatment of 16 patients with metastatic sarcomas, including 11 GISTs. Those investigators used a combination of cisplatin, doxorubicin, mitomycin-C, iodized oil, and PVA. In that patient population, 13% demonstrated a radiologic response and 69% had stable disease. The overall survival rates from the time of embolization were 67% at 1 year, 50% at 2 years, and 40% at 3 years, with a median survival duration of 13 months.

The largest published series to date of patients with metastatic GIST, from Kobayashi and colleagues[20] in 2006, reported on 85 patients with metastatic GIST treated with HACE using cisplatin and PVA or Gelfoam followed in some patients by hepatic arterial infusion of vinblastine. Among these patients, 14% showed a partial response and 74% had stable disease. The overall survival rates in this group were 62% at 1 year, 32% at 2 years, and 20% at 3 years, with a median survival duration of 17.2 months. Patients who had more than five liver metastases and received only one HACE treatment had shorter progression-free survival than did patients with fewer metastases or those who received two or more TACE sessions. Extensive liver involvement, presence of extrahepatic metastases, and progression of liver disease after HACE, were associated with poor overall survival. Concomitant use of imatinib prolonged survival time. Moderate to severe adverse events occurred in 25 of 212 HACE procedures (12%). The complications included pulmonary embolism, cholecystitis, sepsis, severe chest pain, respiratory distress, cardiac event, seizures, and death.

Although many lesions do show a decrease in size after HACE treatment (**Fig. 2**), some lesions may show only tumor necrosis with liquefaction, often without a significant associated lesion shrinkage (**Fig. 3**). If only the tumor size is considered when assessing response rates, as is done with conventional response criteria such as those of the World Health Organization (WHO) and Response Evaluation Criteria in Solid Tumors (RECIST), the true efficacy of the treatment may be substantially

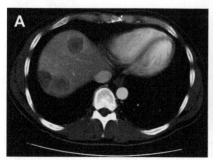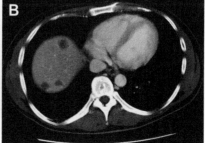

Fig. 2. (*A*) Contrast-enhanced CT (CECT) demonstrates multiple lesions in the right liver. (*B*) CECT obtained after two sessions of HACE shows a decrease in size of the liver lesions.

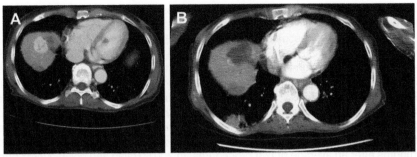

Fig. 3. (A) Contrast-enhanced CT (CECT) demonstrates an enhancing mass in the right liver. (B) CECT obtained after HACE demonstrates a decrease in the density and lack of enhancement of the mass without any appreciable change in lesion size. This patient was considered to have stable disease on the basis of RECIST and a partial response on the basis of modified CT response criteria.

underestimated.[20] To overcome this problem, Choi and colleagues recently devised modified computed tomography (CT) response criteria that use a decrease in tumor size or a decrease in tumor density to define a partial response in GIST treated with imatinib. They reported that their criteria correlate well with the response shown by F-18 fluorodeoxyglucose positron-emission tomography.

Since imatinib is now the first-line treatment for metastatic GIST, transcatheter hepatic arterial embolization and chemoembolization are viable alternatives for patients whose disease has failed to respond to imatinib therapy. This failure is usually a result of the tumor's drug resistance. It is important to mention that sunitinib, the TKI used as second-line therapy for imatinib-resistant GISTs, has no effect on certain imatinib-refractory GISTs having a specific set of gene mutations, such as platelet-derived growth factor A-D842V.[26] HAE and HACE cause destruction of local tumor, irrespective of the mechanism of resistance. There are no series in the literature specifically addressing the role of transcatheter hepatic arterial therapy in the setting

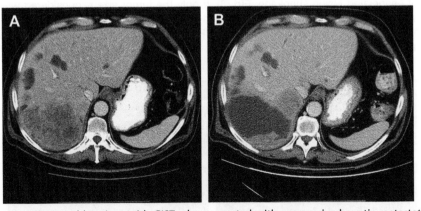

Fig. 4. A 65-year-old patient with GIST who presented with progressive hepatic metastatis while receiving imatinib treatment. (A) Pre-HACE CT demonstrates a large solid mass in the posterior right liver. Note stable cystic metastatic lesions within the rest of the liver. (B) Post-HACE CT demonstrates a decrease in density of the mass.

of imatinib-resistant GIST. At our institution, we performed HAE or chemoembolization in 14 patients with imatinib-resistant GISTs with progressive liver metastasis (Katsuhiro Kobayashi, unpublished data, 2009). Based on RECIST, one patient demonstrated a partial response and 12 patients demonstrated stable disease.

In a multidisciplinary approach, HAE and HACE can be offered to patients with GISTs and liver-dominant metastasis who have primary or acquired resistance to imatinib and are not surgical candidates. Locoregional therapy, including HAE and HACE, is particularly suitable for patients who exhibit an initial response to imatinib in all lesions but later develop progression of focal disease in the liver (**Fig. 4**), such as the case of one solitary lesion that continues to grow. HAE can also be successfully employed in patients who develop intralesional hemorrhage as a complication of imatinib therapy.

SUMMARY

The interventional radiologist plays a limited, but important, role in the diagnosis and management of GISTs. Imatinib mesylate is now established as the first-line therapy for metastatic GIST. The emergence of this targeted agent has dramatically affected the management and outcome of patients with advanced GIST, decreasing the role of locoregional therapy. Nonetheless, RFA remains a potentially curative option for patients whose tumors show a partial response to imatinib with focal residual disease that is not amenable to surgical resection. RFA can also be employed for the control of focal hepatic or peritoneal disease progression in imatinib-resistant patients. The role of hepatic arterial embolization and chemoembolization resides in the treatment of patients with primary or acquired resistance to imatinib who may not be suitable for sunitinib as second-line treatment. In particular, this may be an option for patients who initially exhibit response in all lesions and later show progression in a solitary lesion, or a limited number of lesions, or for patients having a subset of gene mutations that do not respond to sunitinib.

REFERENCES

1. Nilsson B, Bumming P, Meis-Kindblom JM, et al. Gastrointestinal stromal tumors: the incidence, prevalence, clinical course, and prognostication in the preimatinib mesylate era–a population-based study in western Sweden. Cancer 2005;103: 821–9.
2. Trent JC, Benjamin RS. New developments in gastrointestinal stromal tumor. Curr Opin Oncol 2006;18:386–95.
3. Raut CP, Posner M, Desai J, et al. Surgical management of advanced gastrointestinal stromal tumors after treatment with targeted systemic therapy using kinase inhibitors. J Clin Oncol 2006;24:2325–31.
4. Connolly EM, Gaffney E, Reynolds JV. Gastrointestinal stromal tumours. Br J Surg 2003;90:1178–86.
5. DeMatteo RP, Lewis JJ, Leung D, et al. Two hundred gastrointestinal stromal tumors: recurrence patterns and prognostic factors for survival. Ann Surg 2000; 231:51–8.
6. Verweij J, Casali PG, Zalcberg J, et al. Progression-free survival in gastrointestinal stromal tumours with high-dose imatinib: randomised trial. Lancet 2004;364: 1127–34.
7. Van Glabbeke M, Verweij J, Casali PG, et al. Initial and late resistance to imatinib in advanced gastrointestinal stromal tumors are predicted by different prognostic factors: a European Organisation for Research and Treatment of Cancer-Italian

Sarcoma Group-Australasian Gastrointestinal Trials Group study. J Clin Oncol 2005;23:5795–804.

8. Demetri GD, van Oosterom AT, Garrett CR, et al. Efficacy and safety of sunitinib in patients with advanced gastrointestinal stromal tumour after failure of imatinib: a randomised controlled trial. Lancet 2006;368:1329–38.

9. Katz SC, DeMatteo RP. Gastrointestinal stromal tumors and leiomyosarcomas. J Surg Oncol 2008;97:350–9.

10. Dileo P, Randhawa R, Vansonnenberg E, et al. Safety and efficacy of percutaneous radio-frequency (RFA) in patients with metastatic gastrointestinal stromal tumor (GIST) with clonal evolution of lesions refractory to imatinib mesylate. J Clin Oncol 2004;22:9024.

11. Pawlik TM, Vauthey JN, Abdalla EK, et al. Results of a single-center experience with resection and ablation for sarcoma metastatic to the liver. Arch Surg 2006; 141:537–43 [discussion: 543–34].

12. Hasegawa J, Kanda T, Hirota S, et al. Surgical interventions for focal progression of advanced gastrointestinal stromal tumors during imatinib therapy. Int J Clin Oncol 2007;12:212–7.

13. Ahrar K, Gupta S. Hepatic artery embolization for hepatocellular carcinoma: technique, patient selection, and outcomes. Surg Oncol Clin N Am 2003;12:105–26.

14. Nakamura H, Hashimoto T, Oi H, et al. Transcatheter oily chemoembolization of hepatocellular carcinoma. Radiology 1989;170:783–6.

15. Sasaki Y, Imaoka S, Kasugai H, et al. A new approach to chemoembolization therapy for hepatoma using ethiodized oil, cisplatin, and gelatin sponge. Cancer 1987;60:1194–203.

16. Gates J, Hartnell GG, Stuart KE, et al. Chemoembolization of hepatic neoplasms: safety, complications, and when to worry. Radiographics 1999;19:399–414.

17. Perry LJ, Stuart K, Stokes KR, et al. Hepatic arterial chemoembolization for metastatic neuroendocrine tumors. Surgery 1994;116:1111–6 [discussion: 1116–7].

18. Drougas JG, Anthony LB, Blair TK, et al. Hepatic artery chemoembolization for management of patients with advanced metastatic carcinoid tumors. Am J Surg 1998;175:408–12.

19. Kim YH, Ajani JA, Carrasco CH, et al. Selective hepatic arterial chemoembolization for liver metastases in patients with carcinoid tumor or islet cell carcinoma. Cancer Invest 1999;17:474–8.

20. Kobayashi K, Gupta S, Trent JC, et al. Hepatic artery chemoembolization for 110 gastrointestinal stromal tumors: response, survival, and prognostic factors. Cancer 2006;107:2833–41.

21. Mavligit GM, Zukiwski AA, Salem PA, et al. Regression of hepatic metastases from gastrointestinal leiomyosarcoma after hepatic arterial chemoembolization. Cancer 1991;68:321–3.

22. Mavligit GM, Zukwiski AA, Ellis LM, et al. Gastrointestinal leiomyosarcoma metastatic to the liver. Durable tumor regression by hepatic chemoembolization infusion with cisplatin and vinblastine. Cancer 1995;75:2083–8.

23. Gupta S, Johnson MM, Murthy R, et al. Hepatic arterial embolization and chemoembolization for the treatment of patients with metastatic neuroendocrine tumors: variables affecting response rates and survival. Cancer 2005;104: 1590–602.

24. Maluccio MA, Covey AM, Schubert J, et al. Treatment of metastatic sarcoma to the liver with bland embolization. Cancer 2006;107:1617–23.

25. Rajan DK, Soulen MC, Clark TW, et al. Sarcomas metastatic to the liver: response and survival after cisplatin, doxorubicin, mitomycin-C, Ethiodol, and polyvinyl alcohol chemoembolization. J Vasc Interv Radiol 2001;12:187–93.
26. Prenen H, Cools J, Mentens N, et al. Efficacy of the kinase inhibitor SU11248 against gastrointestinal stromal tumor mutants refractory to imatinib mesylate. Clin Cancer Res 2006;12:2622–7.

New Therapeutic Approaches for Advanced Gastrointestinal Stromal Tumors

Neeta Somaiah, MD, Margaret von Mehren, MD*

KEYWORDS

- Gastrointestinal stromal tumor • Nilotinib • Sorafenib
- HSP-90 inhibitors • IGF-1R • Tyrosine kinase inhibitors

Gastrointestinal stromal tumors (GISTs) are the most common type of gastrointestinal (GI) mesenchymal tumors, which as a group are relatively uncommon and constitute less than 1% of all GI tumors. They develop from connective tissue precursors in the GI tract, the interstitial cells of Cajal or its stem cell precursor.[1,2] Management of GISTs has changed dramatically since the discovery that GIST cells express KIT, a receptor tyrosine kinase (RTK) growth factor receptor. CD117 is an antigen on the KIT RTK, the product of the *KIT* proto-oncogene. Staining for CD117 has greatly improved the diagnosis of GIST as it is expressed on 90% to 95% of tumors.[3]

KIT is not only expressed, but is mutated in 85% of cases leading to constitutive activation of the receptor. Mutations are most commonly seen in exon 11, followed in frequency by exons 9, 13, and 17.[4,5] A subset of nonmutated *KIT* tumors have activating mutations in platelet derived growth factor alpha (*PDGFRA*), a related RTK. In *PDGFRA*, mutations are found primarily in exons 12 and 18. Approximately 10% of GISTs do not contain mutations in either *KIT* or *PDGFRA*, the so-called wild-type (WT) GIST. The expression of KIT and the understanding that KIT or PDGFRA are constitutively activated has led to the development of effective targeted therapies using small molecules like imatinib and sunitinib that are tyrosine kinase inhibitors (TKI).

This manuscript was supported in part by NIH grant (CA106588) (to MvM).

Dr. von Mehren has received research support from Novartis and Pfizer and has served on medical advisory boards for Novartis and Infinity Pharmaceuticals.

Department of Medical Oncology, Fox Chase Cancer Center, 333 Cottman Avenue, Philadelphia, PA 19111, USA

* Corresponding author.

E-mail address: margaret.vonmehren@fccc.edu (M. von Mehren).

Hematol Oncol Clin N Am 23 (2009) 139–150

doi:10.1016/j.hoc.2008.12.004

0889-8588/08/$ – see front matter

hemonc.theclinics.com

The therapeutic use of imatinib has revolutionized the treatment in GIST; however, resistance does occur and is a major challenge now. Sensitivity to TKIs such as imatinib and sunitinib depends on the site of mutations in *KIT* and *PDGFRA* (**Table 1**).[6-8] In patients who respond upfront, secondary mutations occur over time, unfortunately leading to resistance. Studies have established the preferred starting dose for imatinib to be 400 mg once daily, with higher dose of 400 mg twice daily recommended as initial therapy only for tumors with exon 9 mutations.[9-12] Dose escalating from low dose over a 4 to 8 week period to the higher dose therapy may lead to fewer severe side effects, which is a significant issue when starting at 400 mg twice daily.[13] Treatment should be continued until progression or intolerance to therapy, given the evidence that disease progression occurs rapidly off of therapy.[14] Here we discuss the approach to advanced GIST, focusing on the different strategies beyond imatinib therapy.

SUNITINIB

For patients who progress on imatinib or are intolerant to imatinib, sunitinib is available as a second-line therapy. Sunitinib is an oral multitargeted receptor TKI; though it binds within the ATP-binding domain of KIT and PDGFRs like imatinib, it is from a different chemical class with presumably different binding affinities. In addition, it also inhibits signaling by all the vascular endothelial growth factor receptor isoforms (VEGF-R1, -R2, -R3), important in tumor angiogenesis, the Fms-like tyrosine kinase-3 receptor (FLT3), and the receptor coded by the ret proto-oncogene. This agent was initially tested using a once daily 50-mg starting dose on a 4-weeks-on followed by 2-weeks-off schedule. After encouraging clinical activity from a phase 1/2 study in patients with imatinib-resistant disease, a phase 3 placebo-controlled trial was conducted by Demetri and colleagues,[15] testing the efficacy and safety of sunitinib after failure of imatinib. In this trial, 312 patients were randomized in a 2-to-1 ratio to sunitinib or placebo and cross over was allowed at the time of progression. The trial was unblinded early when a planned interim analysis revealed a statistically significant longer time to progression (TTP) of 27.3 weeks (95% confidence interval or CI 16–32) with sunitinib, versus 6.4 weeks (95% CI 4.4–10) with placebo. Progression free survival (PFS) and overall survival (OS) were also significantly improved in patients who received sunitinib rather than placebo. Overall objective response rate was similar to previous reports, with 7% showing partial response and 58% with stable disease in the sunitinib group, compared with 0% and 48%, respectively, in the placebo group. Toxicities with this agent are notable for fatigue, hand-foot syndrome, diarrhea, hypertension, mucositis, hypothyroidism, and some serious cytopenias. There have been reports of cardiac toxicity secondary to decrease in ejection fraction and position, necessitating monitoring of cardiac function when using this agent.

Table 1
Potential for disease control with TKI therapy based on site of mutation

TKI	Primary Mutations				Secondary Mutations	
	KIT exon9	*KIT* exon11	*KIT* exon17	*PDGFR* exon18	*KIT* exon13	*KIT* exon14
Imatinib	↓[a]	↑	↓	↓	↓	↓
Sunitinib following Imatinib	↑	ND	↓	↓	↑	↑

↓: Low potential; ↑: High potential; ND: No data.
[a] Less likely to respond to low dose therapy.

The schedule of sunitinib has recently been re-evaluated to test the efficacy and safety of continuous dosing. The rationale for testing a continuous dosing schedule was to avoid the resurgence of metabolic activity in tumors during the 2-week break from sunitinib, as demonstrated by positron emission tomography scan imaging. This phase 2 study of daily sunitinib, at a starting dose of 37.5 mg, showed it was tolerable and with comparable efficacy to the 50-mg starting dose on the conventional schedule.[16] Sixty patients received continuous dosing and the last reported PFS was 27 weeks (95% CI 24–41), with 11% patients experiencing partial response (PR). This schedule is now being tested in a large phase 3 trial compared with high-dose imatinib for patients who have progressed on low-dose imatinib.

Similar to imatinib, there do appear to be selected genotypes that benefit from sunitinib therapy (see **Table 1**). In vitro, the agent is effective against exon 11 mutations. However, the majority of patients treated with sunitinib are patients with tumors containing exon 11 mutations that have progressed after a period of benefit from imatinib. Their tumors typically contain secondary mutations. Sunitinib has activity against those with exon 13 and 14 secondary mutations, with no significant activity against secondary mutations in exon 17. In addition, similar to imatinib, it has minimal activity against primary tumors with *KIT* exon 17 and *PDGFR* exon 18 mutations.[17]

It is not known if the inhibition of angiogenesis by sunitinib contributes to its efficacy over imatinib, as it blocks VEGFR in addition to KIT and PDGFR. An ongoing phase 3 trial of imatinib plus bevacizumab compared with imatinib alone in metastatic GIST patients might shed some light on the added benefit of targeting VEGFR for the treatment of advanced GIST.

Therapies with these TKIs have provided substantial benefits but are not curative in the advanced setting. The role of surgery and other localized therapies have been studied in the metastatic setting, particularly for those patients with focal progression. However for patients with diffuse progression at multiple sites, other options for the imatinib-resistant tumors are needed. This article reviews the role of local therapies as well as discussing additional systemic therapies currently being investigated, including alternative TKI therapies and agents with novel therapeutic targets.

SURGERY AND OTHER LOCAL THERAPIES

Surgery is the mainstay of curative therapy in primary GIST and has traditionally played a palliative role in the advanced disease setting. In the era of targeted therapy, the role for surgery as a part of multimodality management of advanced GISTs has been looked at in small patient series and retrospective studies. One of the rationales for resecting metastases is to eliminate tumors from which drug-resistant clones might develop. The Radiation Therapy Oncology Group studied the role of preoperative imatinib followed by surgery in a phase 2 study in patients with primary locally advanced disease or with recurrent/metastatic disease.[18] Patients with locally advanced disease received 2 years of postoperative imatinib and those with metastatic disease were continued on imatinib until progression. At 2 years, patients with locally advanced disease and metastatic disease had a PFS of 82% (95% CI 68–97) and 73% (95% CI 54–91), respectively, which are encouraging results, suggesting a benefit to surgical debulking in advanced disease.

Studies published from several institutions have demonstrated that surgical debulking might benefit patients with responsive disease or limited progression on kinase inhibitor therapy, but is not beneficial for multifocal progression.[19–22] The largest of these is the retrospective study by Raut and colleagues[20] that evaluated 69 patients who underwent surgery while on kinase inhibitors. The patients were categorized as stable disease, limited progression, or generalized progression, based on their preoperative status. Almost all patients were continued on systemic therapy after surgery. There was a significant association between the preoperative disease status and the extent of residual disease after surgery, as well as the 12-month PFS after surgery. The 12-month PFS was 80%, 33%, and 0% for patients with stable disease, limited progression, and generalized progression, respectively. The complexity of imatinib- and sunitinib-resistance has been demonstrated by molecular studies showing different secondary mutations in several areas within one resected lesion. We now need randomized trials to better evaluate the role of surgery in the metastatic setting and currently studies are being developed to test this in patients who have had disease stabilization on TKI therapy.

Hepatic artery chemoembolization (HACE) and bland embolization has been used for GISTs metastatic to the liver.[23,24] A retrospective series spanning the before- and after-imatinib era showed HACE induced a radiographic durable tumor response and disease stabilization of the liver metastases in 88% of the 85 evaluable patients. The number of embolization treatments, presence of extrahepatic disease, extent of hepatic disease, and use of imatinib were found to have prognostic influence on PFS and OS. Postembolization syndrome with abdominal pain, fever, nausea and vomiting is a common complication with embolization procedures, and therefore may limit the utility of this therapy.

Radio-frequency ablation (RFA) can also be used to treat metastatic lesions within the liver that have focal progression on TKI therapy. Dileo and colleagues[25] reported the outcome with percutaneous CT-guided RFA in nine GIST patients with a single or limited site of progression while on imatinib. Eight of nine patients were treated for progression in the liver, and most of them had a new nodule develop within a pre-existing responding lesion. The procedure was safe and all patients underwent successful ablation of the targeted lesion. Three patients remained stable after RFA after a median follow up of 13.6 months on imatinib, while six progressed systemically after a median of 4.7 months and were increased to 800 mg/day of imatinib, resulting in control for additional 2 to 6 months (median 3.5 months).

ALTERNATE TYROSINE KINASE INHIBITORS

TKIs other than imatinib and sunitinib are being tested for the management of advanced GIST refractory to standard therapy (**Table 2**).

Nilotinib is a second-generation TKI, designed from the crystal structures of imatinib and the ABL-kinase complex and initially developed as a more potent Bcr-Abl inhibitor to override imatinib resistance in chronic myelogenous leukemia.[26] The agent also selectively inhibits phosphorylation of KIT and PDGFR in vitro, and showed promising activity against cell lines expressing exon 13 and 17 double mutants resistant to imatinib.[27] Nilotinib is believed to have enhanced penetration into cells. In addition, encouraging phase 1 data demonstrated stable disease as well as response for this drug in patients with imatinib-resistant GIST when used as a single agent or in combination with imatinib.[28] The recommended doses were nilotinib 400 mg twice daily alone or in combination with imatinib 400 mg daily. Stable disease was noted in 13 out of 18 patients (72%) in the nilotinib-alone arm and 9 of 16 patients (56%) in the combination arm. One patient in each arm experienced a PR, although it should be noted that there were some patients with imatinib-intolerant disease in the nilotinib-alone cohort. Combination therapy was associated with longer duration of therapy and PFS. Grade 3/4 toxicities were seen in 50% of the nilotinib-alone arm and 44% of the combination arm, with the most common adverse effect being grade 3 GI disorders. Dose-limiting

Table 2
OtherTKIs for advanced GIST

Agent	Target in GIST	Phase of Study
Nilotinib	KIT and PDGFR	3
Masitinib	KIT, PDGFR, and FGFR3	3
Sorafenib	RAF kinase, KIT, PDGFR, VEGFR-R2 and R3	2
PKC412	Protein kinase C, KIT, PDGFR, FLT3 and VEGF-R2	1
Vatalanib	KIT, PDGFR, VEGFR-1R and 2R	2
Dasatinib	KIT, PDGFR and SRC family	2
OSI930	KIT and VEGF-R2	1
XL820	KIT, VEGF-R2, and PDGFR	2
AZD2171	KIT, VEGF-R1, R2, R3 and PDGFR	2
MP-470	KIT, PDGFR, c-Met, c-RET and AXL	1
BMS-354,825	KIT, SRC, and PDGFR	2

toxicities noted were hyperbilirubinemia and rash. This study has completed accrual. A phase 3 randomized trial comparing nilotinib versus best supportive care, including continued therapy on imatinib or sunitinib, has completed accrual. Patients on the best supportive-care arm are allowed to cross over to nilotinib at the time of progression. Should the results of this study demonstrate an improved PFS with nilotinib therapy, this may lead to approval of a third-line agent in advanced GIST.

Masitinib mesylate targets c-KIT, PDGFR, and fibroblast growth factor receptor 3 (FGFR3). In vitro, masitinib has demonstrated superior activity to imatinib against WT-*KIT* and *KIT* containing a juxtamembrane region mutation. A phase 1 study of masitinib demonstrated safety and activity, including a complete response in an imatinib-intolerant patient. A multicenter nonrandomized phase 2 trial reported data on 21 imatinib naïve patients with masitinib at 7.5 mg/kg per day.[29] With a median follow up of 9 months, 16 of 21 patients have been on study for greater than 8 weeks. Eleven patients have had a PR (52%), with an additional 8 patients achieving stable disease (38%), and 2 patients demonstrating progressive disease at 8 weeks (10%). One patient with stable disease has subsequently progressed. There were two skin-related grade 3 toxicities and the most frequent side effects were GI-related, with nausea, vomiting, abdominal pain, and diarrhea. These results suggest activity for this agent in GIST. Masitinib will be compared with imatinib in a phase 3 noninferiority trial assessing PFS as the primary study endpoint.

Sorafenib is a raf kinase inhibitor that also has activity against KIT, PDGFR, and VEGFR 2 and 3. In vitro it has demonstrated activity against the imatinib-resistant *PDGFRB* mutation T681 and against cell lines transfected with imatinib-resistant *KIT* mutations, particularly those involving exon 14 T670I and D820Y.[27,30] Single-agent activity of 400-mg oral sorafenib twice daily has been recently reported in patients with imatinib- and sunitinib-resistant GIST.[31] In this phase 2 study, of the 24 subjects evaluable for response, there were 3 subjects with partial responses and 14 with stable disease (disease control rate 71%). The PFS was 23 weeks, similar to that seen in the randomized phase 3 trial of sunitinib, which had a PFS of 27 weeks. Grade 3 toxicities commonly reported include hand-foot syndrome, hypertension, rash, and diarrhea. The role of this agent for refractory disease is of interest and likely will be evaluated further.

PKC412, another broad spectrum kinase inhibitor, has demonstrated preclinical activity against certain *KIT* mutants resistant to imatinib, and the *PDGFRA*-D842V mutation on exon 18 that is relatively insensitive to imatinib and sunitinib.[32–34] Based on in vitro data suggesting synergism with imatinib, PKC412 was evaluated in a phase 1/2 trial in combination with imatinib in patients who developed resistance to imatinib.[35] Unfortunately, strong drug-drug interactions occurred causing a near doubling of PKC steady-state levels and significant decrease in imatinib levels with unusual toxicities and poor efficacy results. After dose modifications to adjust for the interactions, some stabilization of disease was noted in two out of five patients. Increasing thyrotropin levels were noted in four out of seven patients, with one showing clinical hyperthyroidism. The significant pharmacokinetic interactions have limited its tolerability to date, and it is not clear if this agent will be developed further in GIST. Of note, a case report documented disease stabilization with the addition of sirolimus, an mTOR inhibitor to PKC412, after the patient had progressed on imatinib alone and PKC412 alone. This suggests that inhibition of two components of the KIT/PDGFR signaling pathway may be more effective therapeutically (see discussion of the mTOR inhibitor RAD001 below).[36]

Vatalanib (PTK787/ZK222584), a multitargeted TKI, with activity against KIT, PDGFR, and VEGFR-1 and -2, was evaluated in a phase 2 trial in patients with imatinib-resistant GIST.[37] Once daily oral dosing of 1,250 mg produced objective responses as well as stable disease. Of 15 patients enrolled, most of whom had progressed on 800 mg of imatinib daily, two achieved PR with an additional eight having stable disease for 3 or more months, for a clinical benefit rate of 67%. The median TTP was 8.5 months in this small study, which is longer than that reported for sunitinib. The PRs lasted for 9.7 and 20.2+ months and the median duration for stable disease was 10.1 months. Three patients had ongoing favorable responses at the time of analysis. Mutation analysis was available only from two patients: one patient who progressed by week 8 was WT and another with prolonged PR had *KIT* exon 11 deletion. The safety profile was favorable with only two grade 4 events (hypercalcemia and pain), suggesting it may have some advantages over sunitinib. Vatalanib has a short half-life, raising the possibility of better efficacy with twice daily dosing.

Dasatinib is a kinase inhibitor against BCR-ABL, SRC family (SRC, LCK, YES, FYN), c-KIT, EPHA2, and PDGFRB. It is been approved for treatment of imatinib-resistant or intolerant chronic myeloid leukemia and Philadelphia chromosome positive acute lymphoblastic leukemia. Preclinical data by Schittenhelm and colleagues[38] show that dasatinib potently inhibits the kinase activity of WT KIT and juxtamembrane domain mutant KIT isoforms, which are commonly associated with human GISTs. In vitro screening has shown that dasatinib might provide greater benefit than imatinib in certain *KIT* mutants and WT GIST.[27,39] There are ongoing phase 2 studies with dasatinib in front line advanced GIST as well as in imatinib-resistant GISTs.

There are other kinase inhibitors currently being tested in phase 1 or 2 studies, such as XL820, AZD2171, BMS-354,825, MP-470, and OSI930. Some of them have shown activity against secondary mutations resistant to imatinib and sunitinib in vitro. Their role in the management of advanced GIST awaits results from these clinical trials.

NOVEL THERAPEUTIC TARGETS

Other therapeutic strategies being explored in the management of GIST include targeting intracellular components of the KIT/PDGFR signaling pathways, molecules that help maintain the growth factor receptors on the cell surface, or targeting alternative oncogenic pathways (**Table 3**).

Table 3
Agents with novel targets being tested in GIST

Agent	Target	Phase of Trial
RAD001	mTOR inhibitor	2
Perifosine	AKT inhibitor	2
IPI-504	HSP-90 inhibitor	3
CNF2024		2
NVP-AEW541	IGF-1R inhibitor	Preclinical
FR901228	HDAC inhibitor	2
Flavopiridol		1

m-TOR/PI3K/Akt

mTOR is a protein kinase and part of the PI3K/Akt pathway that plays a pivotal role in cell growth and development. Phase 1 and 2 studies have evaluated RAD001, a mammalian target of rapamycin (mTOR) inhibitor, in combination with imatinib.[40] mTOR is downstream of AKT and is important for cell growth and survival. Two cohorts of patients were treated in this study: imatinib-refractory patients and those who had progressed following imatinib and another therapy, usually sunitinib. Patients received imatinib 600 mg and RAD001 2.5 mg per day. PFS was 17.4% and 37.1% in the two cohorts, respectively. Although some activity has been noted, randomized studies will be required to determine RAD001's role compared with other therapeutic strategies available.

In vitro data using cell lines with secondary *KIT* mutations in GIST have demonstrated KIT hyperactivation and imatinib resistance. Therefore, targeting critical downstream signaling proteins, such as PI3K, might be a promising therapeutic strategy in imatinib-resistant GISTs.[41] Current clinical development of MEK and AKT inhibitors is underway and may be useful in combination with TKI therapies. There are currently a few studies testing PI3K inhibitors as single agents. A phase 2 trial is also testing the value of perifosine, a novel AKT inhibitor in combination with imatinib in advanced resistant GIST.

HSP-90

HSP-90 is a novel target in cancer therapeutics. It functions as a molecular chaperone required for the stability and function of several proteins involved not only in normal homeostasis but also in maintaining malignant cell pathways.[42] In particular, it stabilizes oncogenes and receptors, which become more dependent on HSP-90 as they become increasingly mutated. Although directed toward a specific target, HSP-90 inhibitors are capable of inhibiting multiple signaling pathways. This unique feature of inhibiting multiple overlapping survival pathways used by cancer cells give them the potential to circumvent the genetic plasticity that allow these cells to eventually evade the cytotoxic effects of targeted agents.

KIT activation has been shown to be dependent on protein stabilization by HSP-90 and its inhibition, causing degradation of WT KIT and an imatinib resistant mutant in vitro.[43] In GISTs, it is thought that HSP-90 inhibition would result in the loss of the growth signal that emanates from the mutated receptor and, therefore, inhibition of cell growth. Preclinical data have demonstrated activity of HSP-90 inhibitors in cell lines that express either imatinib-sensitive or imatinib-resistant mutations.[44,45]

IPI-504 is a water-soluble HSP-90 inhibitor that has undergone testing in the phase 1 setting in patients progressing on imatinib and sunitinib.[46] Therapy was administered intravenously at test doses of 90 mg/m^2 to 500 mg/m^2 twice weekly for 2 weeks, followed by 1 week off. The dose-limiting toxicities were grade 3 headache and myalgias at the highest-dose level, with 400 mg/m^2 selected for further study. In a group of 36 patients with advanced GIST, there was 1 PR and an additional 24 patients with stable disease. The median TTP was 12 weeks, assessing all dose levels. There was evidence of increased tumor shrinkage in patients receiving higher doses, with one documented partial response. This agent will be entering phase 3 testing in the fall of 2008, comparing it with best supportive care in patients who have progressed following standard therapies. There are additional trials open testing new HSP-90 inhibitors. One of them is CNF2024 in a phase 2 trial in metastatic GIST. Others being tested in solid tumors including GIST are IPI-493, SNX-5422, and AUY-922.

Histone Deacetylases

Epigenetic alterations, such as histone acetylation, have been shown to play a role in the initiation and progression of neoplasm.[47] Histone acetyltransferases and histone deacetylases (HDACs) are two opposing classes of enzymes that tightly control the equilibrium of histone acetylation. This balance plays an important role in the modulation of chromatin structure, chromatin function, and in the regulation of gene expression. An imbalance between these enzyme classes has been associated with carcinogenesis and cancer progression. HDAC inhibitors lead to an accumulation of acetylated histone proteins both in tumor cells and in normal tissues and are able to activate differentiation, to arrest the cell cycle in G1 and G2, and to induce apoptosis in transformed cells. The potential therapeutic value of HDAC inhibitors in treating cancer has been evaluated in clinical trials with a promising outcome.

FR901228 is a new molecule that belongs to this class of therapy and is currently in phase 2 testing for metastatic sarcoma patients including GIST. HDAC inhibitors are also being evaluated in combination with differentiation-inducing agents and cytotoxic drugs for enhanced antitumor activity. Vorinostat (suberoylanilide hydroxamic acid), a HDAC inhibitor, resulted in a prolonged PR for one patient with sarcoma when used along with bortezomib.[48] A similar combination using doxorubicin and flavopiridol is under study in an ongoing phase 1 study for advanced sarcomas including GIST. Results from these will determine if they hold promise for advanced GIST and should be tested further.

Insulin-Like Growth Factor Type I Receptor

Several reports recently have identified the insulin-like growth factor type I receptor (IGF-1R) pathway as a potential pathway in the oncogenesis of GIST. A subset of GISTs lack *KIT* and *PDGFRA* mutations, and these WT-GISTs tend to be less responsive to imatinib-based therapies. Tarn and colleagues[49] reported a higher frequency of aberrant amplification of IGF-1R in WT GISTs and one pediatric WT GIST. In addition, cell lines treated in vitro with an IGF-1R inhibitor (NVP-AEW541), or siRNA silencing of IGF-1R led to cell death and induced apoptosis. The combination of NVP-AEW541 with imatinib induced strong cytotoxicity. A second report highlighted this pathway in pediatric GIST, which usually presents in young girls and commonly are WT.[39] A third report suggested that the presence of ligands for IGF-1R may predict tumor outcome.[50] These reports are exciting and serve as the preclinical data for several upcoming studies testing antibody-based therapies alone or in combination with targeted agents in the treatment of GIST.

SUMMARY

Before the advent of targeted therapy with imatinib, GIST patients who could not be surgically cured had a grim prognosis, as these tumors are resistant to conventional chemotherapy. Apart from its use in first-line treatment of metastatic GIST, imatinib is also being used in the adjuvant setting, where it has shown to prolong recurrence-free survival. Sunitinib is the only approved agent for second-line therapy. Primary and secondary resistance to these agents has been correlated to certain *KIT* and *PDGFRA* mutations. *KIT* and *PDGFRA* mutation testing is being incorporated in some big centers to guide therapy; escalating to high dose imatinib sooner for exon 9 mutations and opting for closer follow-up for mutations unlikely to respond. The challenge for clinicians now is the approach to the patients with disease that is refractory to standard therapies. Several newer TKIs are currently under study and may have a role in the treatment of GIST. Among other agents being studied, the role of HSP-90 inhibitors is intriguing given that it uses a unique therapeutic mechanism. In addition, clinical data for IGF-1R inhibitors is eagerly awaited, given their potential role in patients with WT tumors. In the future, treatment algorithms for GIST patients will change with the identification of tumor subtypes that respond better to one therapy than another.

REFERENCES

1. Wang L, Vargas H, French SW. Cellular origin of gastrointestinal stromal tumors: a study of 27 cases. Arch Pathol Lab Med 2000;124:1471–5.
2. Sircar K, Hewlett BR, Huizinga JD, et al. Interstitial cells of Cajal as precursors of gastrointestinal stromal tumors. Am J Surg Pathol 1999;23:377–89.
3. Fletcher CD, Berman JJ, Corless C, et al. Diagnosis of gastrointestinal stromal tumors: a consensus approach. Hum Pathol 2002;33:459–65.
4. Miettinen M, Lasota J. Gastrointestinal stromal tumors—definition, clinical, histological, immunohistochemical, and molecular genetic features and differential diagnosis. Virchows Arch 2001;438:1–12.
5. Miettinen M, Sobin LH, Sarlomo-Rikala M. Immunohistochemical spectrum of GISTs at different sites and their differential diagnosis with a reference to CD117 (KIT). Mod Pathol 2000;13:1134–42.
6. Lasota J, Corless CL, Heinrich MC, et al. Clinicopathologic profile of gastrointestinal stromal tumors (GISTs) with primary KIT exon 13 or exon 17 mutations: a multicenter study on 54 cases. Mod Pathol 2008;21:476–84.
7. Heinrich MC, Corless CL, Duensing A, et al. PDGFRA activating mutations in gastrointestinal stromal tumors. Science 2003;299:708–10.
8. Hirota S, Ohashi A, Nishida T. Gain-of-function mutations of platelet-derived growth factor receptor alpha gene in gastrointestinal stromal tumors. Gastroenterology 2003;125:660–7.
9. Verweij P, Casali P, Zalcberg P, et al. Progression-free survival in gastrointestinal stromal tumors with high dose imatinib: randomized trial. Lancet 2004;364:1127–34.
10. Blanke CD, Rankin C, Demetri GD, et al. Phase III randomized, intergroup trial assessing imatinib mesylate at two dose levels in patients with unresectable or metastatic gastrointestinal stromal tumors expressing the kit receptor tyrosine kinase: S0033. J Clin Oncol 2008;26:626–32.
11. Debiec-Rychter M, Sciot R, Le Cesne A, et al. KIT mutations and dose selection for imatinib in patients with advanced gastrointestinal stromal tumours. Eur J Cancer 2006;42:1093–103.

12. Heinrich MC, Owzar K, Corless C, et al. Correlation of kinase genotype and clinical outcome in the North American Inter-Group phase III trial of imatinib mesylate for treatment of advanced GI stromal tumor (CALGB 150105). J Clin Oncol 2008;26(33):5360–7.

13. Zalcberg JR, Verjweij J, Casali PG, et al. Outcome of patients with advanced gastro-intestinal stromal tumours crossing over to a daily imatinib dose of 800 mg after progression on 400 mg. Eur J Cancer 2005;41:1751–7.

14. Blay JY, Le Cesne A, Ray-Coquard I, et al. Prospective multicentric randomized phase III study of imatinib in patients with advanced gastrointestinal stromal tumors comparing interruption versus continuation of treatment beyond 1 year: the French Sarcoma Group. J Clin Oncol 2007;25(9):1107–13.

15. Demteri GD, van Oosterom AT, Garett CR, et al. Efficacy and safety of sunitinib in patients with advanced gastrointestinal stromal tumour after failure of imatinib: a randomized controlled trial. Lancet 2006;368:1329–38.

16. George S, Blay JY, Casali PG, et al. Continuous daily dosing (CDD) of sunitinib (SU) in pts with advanced GIST: updated efficacy, safety, PK and pharmacodynamic analysis. J Clin Oncol 2008;26 [abstract 10554].

17. Liegl B, Fletcher JA, Corless CL, et al. Correlation between KIT mutations and sunitinib (SU) resistance in GIST [abstract 92]. In: Programs and abstracts of the 2008 American Society of Clinical Oncology Gastrointestinal Cancer Symposium. Orlando, January 25–27, 2008.

18. Eisenberg BL, Harris J, Blanke C. Phase II trial of neoadjuvant/adjuvant imatinib mesylate (IM) for advanced primary and recurrent operable GI stromal tumor (GIST) – early results of RTOG 0132 [abstract 80]. In: Programs and abstracts of the Society of Surgical Oncology 61st Annual Cancer Symposium. Chicago, March 13–16, 2008.

19. Bonvalot S, Eldweny H, Péchoux CL, et al. Impact of surgery on advanced gastrointestinal stromal tumors (GIST) in the imatinib era. Ann Surg Oncol 2006;13(12):1596–603.

20. Raut C, Posner M, Desai J, et al. Surgical management of advanced gastrointestinal stromal tumors after treatment with targeted systemic therapy using kinase inhibitors. J Clin Oncol 2006;24:2325–31.

21. Rutkowski P, Nowecki Z, Nyckowski P, et al. Surgical treatment of patients with initially inoperable and/or metastatic gastrointestinal stromal tumors (GIST) during therapy with imatinib mesylate. J Surg Oncol 2006;93:304–11.

22. Dematteo R, Maki R, Singer S, et al. Results of tyrosine kinase inhibitor therapy followed by surgical resection for metastatic gastrointestinal stromal tumor. Ann Surg 2007;245:347–52.

23. Kobayashi K, Gupta S, Trent JC, et al. Hepatic artery chemoembolization for 110 gastrointestinal stromal tumors. Cancer 2006;107(12):2833–41.

24. Maluccio MA, Covey AM, Schubert J, et al. Treatment of metastatic sarcoma to the liver with bland embolization. Cancer 2006;107(7):1617–23.

25. Dileo P, Randhawa R, Vansonnenberg E, et al. Safety and efficacy of percutaneous radio-frequency ablation (RFA) in patients with metastatic GIST with clonal evolution of lesions refractory to imatinib mesylate. J Clin Oncol 2004;22 [abstract 9024].

26. Golemovic M, Verstovek S, Giles F, et al. AMN107, a novel aminopyrimidine inhibitor of Bcr-Abl, has in vitro activity against imatinib-resistant chronic myeloid leukemia. Clin Cancer Res 2005;11:4941–7.

27. Guo T, Agaram NP, Wong GC, et al. Sorafenib inhibits the imatinib-resistant KIT-T670I gatekeeper mutation in gastrointestinal stromal tumor. Clin Cancer Res 2007;13:4874–81.

28. Blay JY, Casali PG, Reichardt P, et al. A phase I study of nilotinib alone and in combination with imatinib in patients with imatinib-resistant gastrointestinal stromal tumors (GIST): study update. J Clin Oncol 2008;26 [abstract 10553].
29. Bui BN, Blay J, Duffaud N, et al. Preliminary efficacy and safety results of masitinib, front line in patients with advanced GIST. A phase II study. J Clin Oncol 2007;25 [abstract 10025].
30. Guida T, Anaganti S, Provitera L, et al. Sorafenib inhibits imatinib-resistant KIT and platelet-derived growth factor receptor beta gatekeeper mutants. Clin Cancer Res 2007;13:3363–9.
31. Wiebe L, Kasza K, Maki RG, et al. Sorafenib is active in patients with imatinib and sunitinib-resistant gastrointestinal stromal tumors (GIST): a phase II trial of the University of Chicago Phase II Consortium. J Clin Oncol 2008;26 [abstract 10502].
32. Weisberg E, Wright RD, Jiang J, et al. Effects of PKC412, nilotinib, and imatinib against GIST-associated PDGFRA mutants with differential imatinib sensitivity. Gastroenterology 2006;131:1734–42.
33. Roberts KG, Odell AF, Byrnes EM, et al. Resistance to c-KIT inhibitors conferred by V654A mutation. Mol Cancer Ther 2007;6:1159–66.
34. Debiec-Rychter M, Cools J, Dumez H, et al. Mechanisms of resistance to imatinib mesylate in gastrointestinal stromal tumors and activity of the PKC412 inhibitor against imatinib-resistant mutants. Gastroenterology 2005;128(2):270–9.
35. Reichardt P, Pink D, Lindner T, et al. A phase I/II trial of the oral PKC-inhibitor PKC412 in combination with imatinib mesylate in patients with GIST refractory to imatinib. J Clin Oncol 2005;23 [abstract 3016].
36. Palassini E, Fumagalli E, Coco P, et al. Combination of PKC412 and sirolimus in a metastatic patient with PDGFRA-D842V gastrointestinal stromal tumor (GIST). J Clin Oncol 2008;26 [abstract 21515].
37. Joensuu H, De Braud F, Coco P, et al. A phase II, open-label study of PTK787/ZK222584 in the treatment of metastatic gastrointestinal stromal tumors (GISTs) resistant to imatinib mesylate. Ann Oncol 2008;19:173–7.
38. Schittenhelm MM, Shiraga S, Schroeder A, et al. Dasatinib (BMS-354825), a dual SRC/ABL kinase inhibitor, inhibits the kinase activity of wild-type, juxtamembrane, and activation loop mutant KIT isoforms associated with human malignancies. Cancer Res 2006;66(1):473–81.
39. Agaram NP, Laquaglia MP, Ustun B, et al. Molecular characterization of pediatric gastrointestinal stromal tumors. Clin Cancer Res 2008;14:3204–15.
40. Dumez H, Reichard P, Blay JY, et al.CRAD001C2206 Study Group. A phase I-II study of everolimus (RAD001) in combination with imatinib in patients (pts) with imatinib-resistant gastrointestinal stromal tumors (GIST). J Clin Oncol 2008;26. [abstract 10519].
41. Bauer S, Duensing A, Demetri GD, et al. KIT oncogenic signaling mechanisms in imatinib-resistant gastrointestinal stromal tumor: PI3-kinase/AKT is a crucial survival pathway. Oncogene 2007;26(54):7560–8.
42. Xu W, Neckers L. Targeting the molecular chaperone heat shock protein 90 provides a multifaceted effect on diverse cell signaling pathways of cancer cells. Clin Cancer Res 2007;13:1625–9.
43. Fumo G, Akin C, Metcalfe DD, et al. 17-Allylamino-17-demethoxygeldanamycin (17-AAG) is effective in down-regulating mutated, constitutively activated KIT protein in human mast cells. Blood 2004;103:1078–84.
44. Nakatani H, Kobayashi M, Yin T, et al. STI571 (Glivec) inhibits the interaction between c-KIT and heat shock protein 90 of the gastrointestinal stromal tumor cell line, GIST-T1. Cancer Sci 2005;96:116–9.

45. Bauer S, Yuk LK, Demetri GD, et al. Heat shock protein 90 inhibition in imatinib-resistant gastrointestinal stromal tumor. Cancer Res 2006;66:9153–61.

46. Wagner AJ, Morgan JA, Chugh R, et al. Results from phase 1 trial of IPI-504, a novel HSP90 inhibitor, in tyrosine kinase inhibitor-resistant GIST and other sarcomas. J Clin Oncol 2008;26 [abstract 10503].

47. Santini V, Gozzini A, Ferrari G. Histone deacetylase inhibitors: molecular and biological activity as a premise to clinical application. Curr Drug Metab 2007;8(4): 383–93.

48. Schelman WR, Kolesar J, Schell K, et al. A phase I study of vorinostat in combination with bortezomib in refractory solid tumors. J Clin Oncol 2007;25. [abstract 3573].

49. Tarn C, Rink L, Merkel E, et al. Insulin-like growth factor 1 receptor is a potential therapeutic target for gastrointestinal stromal tumors. Proc Natl Acad Sci U S A 2008;105:8387–92.

50. Braconi C, Bracci R, Bearzi I, et al. Insulin-like growth factor (IGF) 1 and 2 help to predict disease outcome in GIST patients. Ann Oncol 2008. [Epub ahead of print].

Index

Note: Page numbers of article titles are in **boldface** type.

A

Ablation, radiofrequency, of GIST metastatic to liver, 130–131
Advanced disease, in GIST, new approaches for, **139–150**
    alternate tyrosine kinase inhibitors, 142–144
    novel therapeutic targets, 144–146
        histone deacetylases, 146
        HSP-90, 145–146
        insulin-like growth factor type 1 receptor, 146
        m-TOR/PI3K/Akt, 145
    sunitinib, 140–141
    surgery and other local therapies, 141–142
  treatment of, 73–75
Age, in familial GIST syndrome, 2
Animal models, of familial GIST syndrome, 6–7
Anthracyclines, cardiotoxicity attributable to, in patients with GIST, 97–98

B

Biologic therapy, surgery and, for GIST primary and synchronous liver metastases, 121–123
Biopsy, of GIST, interventional radiology in, 130

C

Cardiovascular effects, of tyrosine kinase inhibitors used for GIST, **97–107**
    cardiotoxicity of, 97–98
    imatinib mesylate, 99–101
    practical approach to prevention of cardiotoxicity, 103–104
    promise of molecularly targeted therapy, 98–99
    sunitinib malate, 101–102
Carney triad, GIST in, 7, 17
Carney-Stratakis syndrome, GIST in, 7, 17
  succinate dehydrogenase in, 28
CD34, as immunohistochemical marker in diagnosis of GIST, 54–57
Chemical therapy, surgery and, for GIST primary and synchronous liver metastases, 121–123
Chemoembolization, hepatic arterial, for GIST metastatic to liver, 131–135
Clinical features, of GIST, 4–5, 17–25, 50–51, 71
Computed tomography (CT), of GIST, 36–41
    initial evaluation, 36–37
    response evaluation, 37–40
    surveillance, 40
    technical limitations, 41

Hematol Oncol Clin N Am 23 (2009) 151–158
doi:10.1016/S0889-8588(09)00024-0
hemonc.theclinics.com

Moving?

Make sure your subscription moves with you!

To notify us of your new address, find your **Clinics Account Number** (located on your mailing label above your name), and contact customer service at:

E-mail: elspcs@elsevier.com

800-654-2452 (subscribers in the U.S. & Canada)
314-453-7041 (subscribers outside of the U.S. & Canada)

Fax number: 314-523-5170

Elsevier Periodicals Customer Service
11830 Westline Industrial Drive
St. Louis, MO 63146

*To ensure uninterrupted delivery of your subscription, please notify us at least 4 weeks in advance of move.

ELSEVIER

Printed and bound by CPI Group (UK) Ltd, Croydon, CR0 4YY

03/10/2024

01040450-0017